OTHER BOOKS BY NATHAN PRITIKIN

The Pritikin Program for Diet and Exercise

The Pritikin Permanent Weight-Loss Manual

The Pritikin Promise

BY NATHAN PRITIKIN AND ILENE PRITIKIN

The Official Pritikin Guide to Restaurant Eating

Nathan Pritikin

DIET FOR RUNNERS

A FIRESIDE BOOK

PUBLISHED BY SIMON & SCHUSTER, INC.
NEW YORK

Copyright © 1985 by Pritiken International, a California Corporation
All rights reserved
including the right of reproduction
in whole or in part in any form
First Fireside Edition, 1986
Published by Simon & Schuster, Inc.
Simon & Schuster Building
Rockefeller Center
1230 Avenue of the Americas
New York, New York 10020
FIRESIDE and colophon are registered trademarks of Simon & Schuster, Inc.
Manufactured in the United States of America

10   9   8   7   6   5   4

Library of Congress Cataloging in Publication Data

ISBN: 0-671-55623-1 (Pbk.)
ISBN: 0-671-60071-0

— ACKNOWLEDGMENTS —

It has been my good fortune to have had the assistance of a very able team in writing this book. Nan Bronfen Smith, Director of Nutrition Research for the Pritikin Research Foundation, was responsible for much of the library research and manuscript preparation. Her good judgment, talents, and unstinting efforts are reflected throughout. Ilene Pritikin, my wife, prepared the material on the food plan and organized the excellent recipe section.

Miles H. Robinson, M.D., helped edit the manuscript, and, in addition, wrote the chapter entitled "Runners' Deaths." Tricia Thompson typed much of the manuscript and made many good suggestions, and Nell Taylor, my secretary, compiled the recipe index, typed, and edited.

The recipe section of this book would not have been possible without the contributions of our chef, Esther Taylor, who worked closely with my wife to test, adapt, and create recipe after recipe. Some of the recipes tested were sent to us by chefs at the Pritikin Longevity Center in Santa Monica, California, and Downingtown, Pennsylvania. We are grateful to them and others whose culinary inspirations found their way into the recipe section. My thanks, also, to Janet Trent, who assisted in editing the recipes.

Scientific drawings by Nell Taylor are reprinted from *The Pritikin Promise*.

NATHAN PRITIKIN

TO ILENE PRITIKIN

- a dedicated runner
- 25 years old (don't believe her birth certificate that says over 60)
- my coauthor
- my inspiration

CONTENTS

FOREWORD

The appalling phenomenon of runners' deaths has evoked much controversy about the safety of running, even for people in apparently excellent health. There is compelling evidence that these deaths are due to the fact that most runners still follow the average American diet. I discussed this point in a previous book, *The Pritikin Promise: 28 Days to a Longer, Healthier Life,* but I felt there was a real need for a more extended treatment of the subject of diet as it affects runners. Hence this book. You will find another important feature in this book—a special convenience diet developed especially for runners, on which they can "carbohydrate-load" safely at every meal.

PART ONE

NUTRITION AND YOUR HEALTH

1

How the Pritikin Diet Can Help You

Why should you—a healthy person—a runner, no less—bother to change the way you eat?

The sad news is that, in all likelihood, you're not as healthy as you may think. If you are over 20 years old and have been on an American diet all your life, you're undoubtedly not healthy at all. In fact, statistics suggest you are probably well on your way to suffering severe heart disease.

Here is why:

The heart is a muscle and requires blood to work. Only three coronary arteries, each as thin as a pencil, supply all the blood to your heart. If these arteries become clogged with cholesterol deposits or "boils" from too much fat and cholesterol in your diet, they will narrow or close so that the volume of blood flowing to your heart diminishes. So even though your heart muscle is strong because you run, .you are probably forming fatty deposits in the vessels sup-

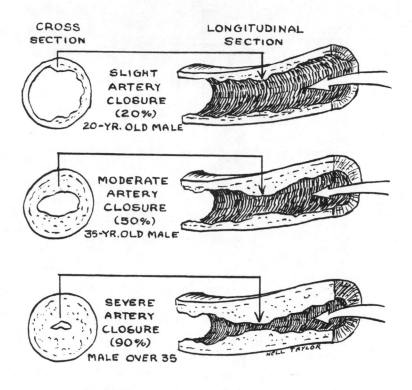

THREE STAGES OF PROGRESSIVE
HEART DISEASE

plying that muscle, which means you probably have heart disease.

Let's look at the odds.

Are you male and 20? In all likelihood your three coronary arteries average 20 percent closure. You are in the early stages of heart disease, even though you feel fine. For now.

Are you female and 30? The odds are that you're as sick as that 20-year-old man. You lag ten years behind men on the road to heart disease, but you'll catch up after menopause.

Are you male and 35? Your coronary arteries are likely 50 percent blocked, although you still feel well. Even if all three coronaries are 65 percent closed, it is possible to pass the most vigorous stress treadmill test and be told that you are very healthy. Until at least one of your coronary arteries is 90–100 percent closed, you will have no symptoms. Then you might notice some chest pressure when you exercise. When that happens you are a prime candidate for a heart attack and you could suddenly die while running. You might remember that Arthur Ashe, world-class tennis player, had a serious heart attack at 36. He had no idea he had heart disease until one of his coronary arteries closed completely and he began to feel pressure in his chest. Fortunately his condition was diagnosed in time. Ashe had bypass surgery and is doing well today. Others have not been as lucky.

So don't wait until your condition is serious enough to be diagnosed as heart disease. By that time your arteries will be so narrowed with cholesterol deposits that you could die without warning from heart disease. It happens to 350,000 Americans every year. And most of them were given a clean bill of health at their most recent physical examination.

WHAT DOCTORS CAN—AND CAN'T—TELL YOU

Doctors cannot accurately predict whether you will have a heart attack. They can only give you odds based on risk factors, such as cholesterol level, blood pressure, smoking, weight, activity, and heredity. They can make predictions on the basis of electrocardiograph (EKG) and stress (treadmill) testing. However, even stress testing is only 75 percent accurate.

The most reliable laboratory test in determining the probability of death from heart disease is the blood test to measure the level of serum cholesterol. Still, it is only 85 percent accurate.

In the end, the amount of cholesterol in your *diet* is the only reliable indicator of whether you have, or will have, serious heart disease. We have conclusive evidence for this from a comprehensive and well-controlled study done by the National Institutes of Health (NIH). The researchers found that when you decrease the cholesterol in your *diet* enough to drop your *blood* cholesterol one percent, it results in about a two percent decrease in your risk of heart disease if your cholesterol is above 265. Where does the Pritikin diet fit with all of this? Studies show the Pritikin diet promotes a 25 percent drop in blood cholesterol in only three weeks. Pretty impressive! Every year one million Americans die from some form of heart disease.

The statistics are shocking, and so are some of the facts supporting them. Because of our high fat American diet, our arteries start closing in our teens. In 1953 Dr. William Enos reported on evidence gained from autopsies performed on 300 American soldiers killed in the Korean War. Their average age had been 22. Seventy-seven percent of the men showed evidence of coronary disease from minimal eccentric thickening to complete occlusion of one or more of the three main coronary arteries.

Nine of these young men had complete closure of one or more of their main coronary arteries! Dr. Enos blamed the artery closure on the American diet. He performed autopsies on Japanese males 20–30 years old who had been on a typically low-fat diet, and he found none with any significant artery closures.

Now, 30 years later, because of the increasing popularity of fast-food chains and their high-fat, cholesterol-laden foods, physicians agree that virtually *all* 20-year-olds have narrowing of their arteries. Unfortunately, most young people feel reasonably well and see no need to change their diets. They often respond to suggestions that they make dietary changes with:

"So I'll live 20 years less—but I'll enjoy living!"
"What's life without a five-egg omelette?"
"No one is going to tell me what to eat!"
"I'm addicted to candy bars."
"I have to have ten cups of coffee to get through the day."
"My grandfather ate eggs, smoked, and drank whiskey, and lived to be 132 years old."

They seem unable—or unwilling—to consider two things:
1. How they will feel in ten years' time if they continue on their present course; and
2. How much better they could be feeling and functioning right now.

With the Pritikin Program everyone, regardless of age, will notice dramatic changes in a few weeks or less. Here are some of the benefits you—a healthy person—can derive from the program.

FEEL LESS FATIGUED

Why are you so exhausted after lunch; on weekends; when you get home from work at night? Naturally, you feel tired if you have not had enough sleep. But lack of sleep is easily remedied, and it is *not* the most common cause of lethargy. Fatigue is most often caused by an inadequate supply of oxygen to our muscles and brain cells.

If you have a fit of yawning, deep breathing will increase your oxygen supply slightly for a few seconds. If you want to dramatically increase the oxygen available to your body's cells on a permanent basis, you will have to adhere to a diet low in fat. Tired blood is low-oxygen blood, and low-oxygen blood is too high in fats. Here's why: Blood is a watery substance densely packed with different types of cells, sugar, proteins, amino acids, fats, salts, vitamins, hormones, and many other substances. But the major component of blood is red blood cells—five million per cubic millimeter (a volume about half that of a grain of rice). The red cells resemble life preservers with a thin membrane stretched across the hole. They are filled with hemoglobin, which carries the oxygen throughout the body.

The arteries carrying the blood become ever smaller as they approach the tissues to be nourished.

The red cells pass, one at a time, through the tiniest vessels and each one moves very close to the tissue cell it nourishes with oxygen. But after a fatty meal, the blood is greasy for many hours and, as a result, the red cells and other blood cells stick together. The more they stick together the less able they are to pass through the capillaries. Therefore, some tissue is undernourished.

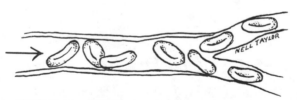

NORMAL RED CELLS EASILY PASS
INTO TINY CAPILLARIES

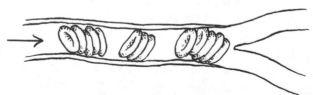

CLUMPED RED CELLS HAVE DIFFICULTY
PASSING INTO THE CAPILLARIES

When our brain and muscles become oxygen-deprived, we feel both physically and mentally tired. A low-fat diet will wake up both body and mind, because the red cells will carry less fat and more oxygen and find it easier to make deliveries to the tissue cells.

FEEL MORE ENERGETIC

Our bodies need plenty of oxygen to convert food into energy. Restricting the fat in the diet allows more oxygen into our tissue cells, so we will feel more energetic. You have to rid your system of the excess fat and aerate it to feel your most alive, alert, and energetic.

IMPROVE ENDURANCE AND PERFORMANCE

If you are already active in sports, the Pritikin Program will increase your endurance and enhance your performance. Only a regular diet of meals high in complex carbohydrates will provide optimal levels of energy at all times.

Over the years, carefully controlled studies of skiers and subjects riding stationary bicycles have demonstrated that people on high-carbohydrate diets have more endurance than those on a high-protein diet. These studies show that the benefits of the high-carbohydrate diet include improved work performance and reaction time, increased altitude tolerance, and better control of blood sugar levels.

LESS RISK OF DEGENERATIVE DISEASES

The Pritikin Program can greatly reduce your chances of developing heart disease, diabetes, and several types of cancer, depending upon how much at risk you were to begin with. This is determined by evaluation of risk factors. Different diseases are associated with different risk factors, and of course, different diseases have many risk factors in common. Among the risk factors associated with the most prevalent degenerative diseases are high blood pressure, high or low blood sugar, high levels of cholesterol and/or triglycerides in the blood, high levels of uric acid, smoking, excessive alcohol consumption, and being overweight. By reducing your risk factors, you will be considerably less likely to develop these diseases.

NO MORE CONSTIPATION

Fiber in our food absorbs several times its weight in water, giving bulk to the intestinal contents and moving waste products through the colon. Because the Pritikin diet contains ample amounts of natural fiber, it prevents the common problem of "irregularity." Americans spend millions of dollars each year on laxatives. The expense, discomfort, and disorders that can be caused by constipation, such as hemorrhoids, varicose veins, and diverticular disease, can be prevented by a sensible diet consisting mainly of foods as grown.

BETTER MENTAL ACUITY

In 1977, 31 patients at the Longevity Center in California were tested before starting the Pritikin diet and exercise program and again after three weeks to determine the effect of the program on mental acuity and personality. The pilot results indicated improvement in both these areas.

EASIER MENSTRUAL PERIODS

Dietary fats and cholesterol affect reproductive functions. Girls on a high-fat diet start menstruating at an earlier age, and women reach menopause at a later age. Prostaglandin production, which is affected by dietary fat, increases the amount of flow during menstrual periods, the length of the period, and cramping. Women on the low-fat Pritikin diet have had dramatic results with these problems, and they have also found that regular exercise such as running reduces menstrual cramping and low back pain.

LONGER LIFE

Researchers have been demonstrating for more than 50 years that restricting the food intake of animals ranging from one-celled creatures to humans results in a lengthened life span. Unrestricted feeding, on the other hand, promotes increased rate of growth, a greater amount of body fat, earlier onset of degenerative diseases, and premature death.

More recent studies have shown that it is not only the quantity of food but its composition that affects the aging process. For instance, if a diet is high in protein, it has to be hypocaloric (or low-caloric) to effect increased longevity, but if it is high in carbohydrates, the caloric content is of no consequence. A diet low in protein (8 percent) and high in carbohydrates (83 percent) when fed to rats in unrestricted amounts was as effective as when higher-protein diets were fed to them on a restricted basis. The more protein and fat in the diet, the shorter the life span. More carbohydrates increased the life span, sometimes almost doubling it even if calories were not restricted.

We have no reason to believe that the composition of the diet will not have the same type of effect on humans. If it does, then eating a high-carbohydrate diet will enable us to live healthier, more enjoyable, and longer lives.

Many diet book authors are rapidly working in the direction of the Pritikin dietary guidelines, and most new cookbooks today feature low-fat, low-cholesterol, low-sodium, sugarless, or vegetarian recipes. They're recommending more use of complex-carbohydrate foods, such as beans, grains and grain products, and vegetables. They're going with the tide, and they are not the only ones. Government agencies are moving in the same direction.

In 1976 and 1977, Senator George McGovern presided over the Select Committee on Nutrition and Human Needs. Typical of the testimony before the committee was that of Harvard School of Public Health professor Mark Hegsted. He stated that the increased amount of fatty, cholesterol-rich, and refined foods in the diet was responsible for the high rates of heart disease, hypertension, certain forms of cancer, and obesity. He said, "We cannot afford to temporize. We have an obligation to inform the public of the current state of knowledge and to assist the public in making the correct food choices. To do less is to avoid our responsibility."

The committee subsequently published its "Dietary Goals." The recommendations approached those of the Pritikin Research Foundation. They urged Americans to increase significantly their intake of carbohydrates; decrease the amount of sugar in the diet; eat less meat, butter, and eggs; and in general decrease dietary fat (both saturated and unsaturated), cholesterol, and salt.

In his 1979 report to the American people the surgeon general admonished us, "You, the individual, can do more for your own health and well-being than any doctor, any hospital, any drug, any exotic medical advice." This report also approaches the Pritikin dietary guidelines in its recommendations to eat more complex carbohydrates and less fat, cholesterol, salt, and sugar. The American Diabetes Association, in its earlier years, used to recommend that 30 percent of the calories in the diet of diabetics come from carbohydrates, but recently the complex-carbohydrate allotment was increased to 60 percent. The latest, safest, most efficient way to normalize carbohydrate metabolism in both diabetics and nondiabetics is with the high-carbohydrate, high-natural-fiber diet.

Some organizations are still sitting on the fence. The U.S. Department of Agriculture, for instance, was quite unspecific in its 1981 publication on diet, saying, "Avoid too much fat, cholesterol, sugar, and sodium." Of course, too much is too much, but the publication doesn't tell us how much that is. It doesn't tell us whether we should eat less than we eat now or whether "too much" means even more than the quantities of those substances the average American already consumes. There is so much scientific evidence demonstrating the risks we incur by eating animal products indiscriminately that the department does at least mention that "too much" fat and cholesterol can be harmful. It is my hope that as the current of nutritional enlightenment becomes stronger and stronger, even the U.S. Department of Agriculture will be forced to dedicate itself to the task of improving the supply of safe wholesome food for all Americans.

If these benefits of the Pritikin Program aren't enough, we can also state unequivocally that you will look better and younger than ever *and* save money! The average family of four saves $1,500 per year on groceries with our program.

Let's take a look now at how the Pritikin Program works to make you healthier than ever.

2

High-Protein Diets, Carbohydrate Loading, and Other Nutritional Dangers

The Pritikin diet is ideal for runners, hikers, bikers, mountain climbers, spelunkers, and other outdoor sports fans. If you're active in sports, you need the same nutrients as sedentary people. Your body will require some of the vitamins and minerals in slightly larger amounts, but the Pritikin diet will supply them even if you aren't eating a greater quantity of food to provide the extra calories you need. You do need to increase the amount of carbohydrates you eat, but you don't need additional fat or protein. Scientific studies have shown that on a diet high in complex carbohydrates, athletes have up to three times the endurance of those on the conventional high-protein, high-fat diets.

PROTEIN

Many athletes and body builders believe they should eat more protein. This is not the case, however. Dave Scott sets a new record each time he wins the Hawaii Ironman Triathlon, which he's done for the past three years—on a diet high in starchy foods. Many people were astonished to learn that on a diet low in animal protein, the "Ironman" could survive, not to mention break world records. Their skepticism was in large part due to the prevalence of myths regarding nutrition and athletic performance—mainly the big protein myth.

You do not have to eat large quantities of protein to build muscles! Think of the bull who grows big and strong eating nothing but grass all day. Unfortunately, the "eat muscle to make muscle" type of reasoning still motivates some weight lifters who eat diets high in animal foods and take protein-powder supplements to promote muscle development. The problem is, the extra protein goes to fat—not to muscle.

Even on a strict vegetarian diet that includes no eggs or dairy products, if an athlete eats enough food to maintain his/her weight, there will be more than enough protein for muscle growth and maintenance. Excess protein will go to fat—unless the diet is deficient in carbohydrates, in which case the protein will be used inefficiently as a fuel source to provide energy.

To build muscle, sufficient calories—primarily from carbohydrates—small amounts of protein, and vigorous strenuous activity are needed. You simply cannot substitute protein supplements for proper diet and hard work. In order to enlarge and strengthen muscles, you have to stress them—increase the demand on them to produce energy. Enzymes in the tiny "organs," or mitochondria, of muscle cells provide the energy for physical work, and as the demand on the cells to produce energy increases, your muscles grow by forming more and bigger mitochondria. Prolonged strenuous exercise is the only way to get bigger muscles. Forget about the extra protein and get to work!

The Pritikin diet is ideal not only for people engaged in endurance sports but for body builders as well. Fifteen-year-old John Wardell is a case in point. Four years ago John put down his baseball mitt and picked up a set of weights. With his change in sport came a change in diet. His father had been a firm advocate of the Pritikin Diet, so John gave it a try and has been on it ever since.

On March 31, 1984, John won the teenage division of the NPC Tri-State Body Building Championships in New York City.

John did not need to eat a lot of protein to increase muscle mass. He simply ate sensibly and did a lot of lifting. His diet and training program resulted in some mighty impressive muscles.

Not only does extra protein not make bigger and better muscles, it can actually be extremely dangerous for athletes. As you will understand by now, we need small amounts of protein and fat for our body tissues, enzymes, and hormones; but the fuel source for our *energy* requirements should be carbohydrate—a clean-burning fuel. When carbohydrate is converted to energy, only carbon dioxide and water remain, and our bodies excrete these chemicals quite easily. Ideally, our entire energy or calorie requirement should come from carbohydrates.

When there is adequate dietary carbohydrate to provide this energy, excess protein, fat, and carbohydrate will be stored as potential energy in the form of fat in the adipose tissues throughout the body. In the absence of sufficient carbohydrate foods, fats and proteins will be converted to the energy needed to keep the body functioning—breathing, digesting, regulating its temperature, and so on.

The problem is that in order for protein to be digested and converted to energy or stored as fat, it has to rid itself of its ammonia molecules, which are left as waste products. Because ammonia is toxic to the cells and difficult to eliminate, we say that protein does not burn clean. As the process continues, two ammonia molecules are joined to form urea. This is less toxic than ammonia, but harmful enough to require large amounts of water to dilute its toxicity so that it can be excreted without damage to the kidneys. High-protein diets are therefore very dehydrating.

Dehydration is of great concern to athletes, who lose enormous quantities of water through perspiration. The body keeps from overheating via perspiration, and evaporation of moisture on the surface of the skin has a cooling effect. Thus the body keeps its internal temperature from increasing too much during strenuous exercise. However, when you are dehydrated, your evaporative cooling mechanism is adversely affected, and you may suffer heatstroke, which can be—and too often is—fatal to athletes exercising strenuously in hot weather.

In addition, too much protein causes minerals like calcium to leave the bones in order to neutralize the acids formed in protein metabolism. We believe this to be a principal cause of weak or thin bones (osteoporosis)—epidemic in the United States for those over 50 years old.

And finally, excess protein can have detrimental effects on your performance and endurance. A number of studies have shown that on a mixed diet one has greater endurance than on a high-protein diet; but on a high-carbohydrate diet, athletes have *three times* the endurance they have on a high-protein diet. "Carbs" are the fuel of winners. So it is not really so surprising that the best-performing athletes in the Hawaii Ironman Triathlon were those on the Pritikin diet.

Carbohydrates provide greater endurance for other species as well. Carnivorous animals can run with great speed but their endurance is minimal. Cats, for instance, have the ability to run faster than almost any other animal. The carcal lynx and the cheetah have been clocked at up to 65 mph, but only for short distances. Cats are also renowned for the inordinate amount of time they spend sleeping. However, herbivores, which make up the bulk of the animal kingdom, have far greater endurance. Giraffes and racehorses can not only run 45 mph, but can sustain this speed for long periods of time.

The endurance of man and pig, two of the few omnivorous animals, lies midway between that of the meat- and the plant-eaters.

FATS

Fats are a necessary part of our makeup because energy can be stored in a concentrated form in fat cells. During exercise, large amounts of both carbohydrate and fat from the storage depots provide us with energy. Therefore, some athletes believe they need to eat a lot of fat. But a higher proportion of our energy comes from fat when we're at rest than when we're exercising. The idea that athletes need to eat more fat resembles the myth that in order to be brave you have to eat the heart of a lion; or that in order to make muscle you have to eat muscle. In actuality, the "fat" or fatty acids we burn for fuel do not come directly from our food. They are liberated from fats in the adipose (fat) tissue, and the fats in this tissue have come from carbohydrates and proteins as well as fats. It is actually preferable that very little of this fat be derived from fatty foods. In fact, we can get most of the fat we need from whole grains. (Be aware, though, that the essential fatty acids have been removed from refined flour.)

Fats are composed of three fatty acids attached to a short skeleton, called glycerol. Fats are also called triglycerides, which means "three fatty acids." In order to be stored in the cells of adipose tissue, fatty acids must become part of a triglyceride. Subsequently, the triglycerides in the adipose tissue must be broken down into fatty acids before being released into the blood and transported to the muscle cells to be burned for energy. Adipose tissue is like Grand Central Station. Free fatty acids are constantly breaking away from the triglyceride (fat) molecules in the adipose-tissue station to travel in the bloodstream. Those not used for energy return and become part of a triglyceride so they can enter the station again to be stored until needed.

CARBOHYDRATES

The typical American diet doesn't provide enough carbohydrate for athletes in hard training. As you now know, most of the calories of sedentary people should come from carbohydrates, and athletes need an even larger percentage of carbohydrates.

Carbohydrate is the main fuel for endurance, and it can be the limiting factor if your diet is deficient in carbohydrates. Some ardent athletes, especially runners, adhere to a potentially dangerous and misnamed practice called carbohydrate loading. This is their reasoning: Because only a small amount of carbohydrate is stored in muscle cells in the form of glycogen, they believe they should increase the amount of this potential energy. Endurance athletes will therefore exercise themselves to exhaustion seven days prior to a competitive event. For the next three days they curtail severely the amount of carbohydrate in their diets by subsisting mainly on high-fat animal products—dairy foods, meat, and eggs. This causes depletion of glycogen in the muscles. During the next three days, they eat high-carbohydrate meals in order to load their muscles with glycogen. After the three-day depletion phase, the muscles overcompensate and take up an abnormally large amount of glycogen.

There are several dangers in this scheme. First, during the depletion phase of carbohydrate loading, the low-carbohydrate diet causes large amounts of fat to circulate in the blood. Should the athlete have heart disease, this could precipitate a heart attack. It can even cause cardiac irregularities in highly trained individuals without preexisting heart problems.

Also, carbohydrate loading causes enormous amounts of

glycogen to be stored in all the muscles that have been worked to exhaustion during the depletion phase —not only the leg muscles, but the heart muscles as well. Glycogen is stored with three to four times its own weight in water. You can well imagine how difficult it will be for a heart so engorged to function properly.

Carbohydrate loading can cause prostatitis, or swelling of the prostate gland, resulting in very painful urination. It can also lead to potassium depletion and a possible heatstroke during the event. Metabolizing fats in the absence of sufficient carbohydrates can also result in the formation of ketones— toxic substances which, when excreted, can cause dehydration damage to the kidneys. Less dangerous, but certainly worth considering, is the fact that the weight of the glycogen and the water with which it is stored will make the athlete's legs feel heavy. So much glycogen can be taken up that the muscle tissue can rupture, reducing performance.

The best way to improve endurance and performance is to adhere to the Pritikin diet. That way, you are carbohydrate loading—safely—all the time. Your muscles will have an optimal amount of glycogen without the dangerous side effects of depletion/engorging carbohydrate loading.

On the average, carbohydrates make up 50 percent of the calories in the typical American diet. Studies by Dr. David Costill, at Ball State University in Indiana, show that on the 50 percent carbohydrate diet, it takes three days after strenuous exercise to restore the proper glycogen levels, but that it takes only one day if you're on a 70 percent carbohydrate diet.

Thus when only half of your calories come from carbohydrates, you can't perform at your best for three days following competitive events or heavy training. On the Pritikin diet, however, you're ready to do your best after a single day of rest. After one day on a high–complex-carbohydrate diet, the muscles are fully loaded with glycogen.

Just remember that for the most part it's complex carbohydrates or starches rather than simple sugars you should be eating. For a while it was popular among runners to drink expensive sugar beverages for "quick energy." The latest rage among athletes seeking a magic bullet to give them an edge on the competition is fructose. Use of fructose, an extravagant health food store item, has spawned a lot of misleading ideas—that it increases endurance, causes weight loss, and is beneficial as a substitute for regular sugar in the diet of diabetics. Scientific investigation has not found these claims to be valid.

Ordinary table sugar is half glucose and half fructose. Because fructose is absorbed more slowly, it can cause stomach bloating, cramps, gas, and diarrhea. Fructose also raises blood fats to a significant degree, which is dangerous for people with heart disease and for runners because fats in the blood prevent optimal oxygen delivery to the working muscles.

VITAMINS

In spite of numerous studies disproving any ergogenic, or work-enhancing, effect of vitamin supplements, some athletes continue to believe in such effects. Dr. D. L. Cooper, a physician at the 1972 Olympics, said, "Vitamins need to be mentioned as another subject of the 'great drug myths.' We must remember that vitamins act primarily as catalytic agents and are not metabolized. If a person eats a balanced diet of fresh, well-prepared food, he is getting all the vitamins his body can use. . . . There are many salesmen in this country and many gullible people who are victimized financially by vitamin 'pushers.' Americans excrete the most expensive urine in the world because it is loaded with so many vitamins!"

Vitamin E is the vitamin most often taken by athletes to improve their performance and increase their endurance. The fact is that large amounts may actually reduce endurance, and in some people cause weakness and fatigue.

In a 50-day double-blind study of ice hockey players in Canada, scientists set out to determine whether vitamin E might give just that little edge of extra endurance that athletes need toward the end of a game. Twenty hockey players were paired off according to what is called oxygen uptake, a measurement of their maximum endurance. One group received 1,200 IU of vitamin E and the other group only a placebo. They were tested on treadmills before and after the 50 days. Those taking the vitamin E increased the maximum amount of oxygen they could consume by 10 percent. Those on the placebo increased the maximum amount of oxygen they could consume by 30 percent. The researcher, Dr. Good, an associate professor in the Department of Physiology, University of Toronto, wrote, "One facetious observation might be that placebo may result in greater improvement than vitamin E."

Vitamin C has also been tested to determine whether supplementation would have ergogenic effects. Two groups of 20 young (average age: 24.5) physical education majors were given treadmill tests before and after a five-day ingestion of either two grams of vitamin C or a placebo. The double-blind test showed no significant difference between those who took vitamin C and those on the placebo.

The B vitamins act along with enzymes as coenzymes, or catalysts in the conversion of food, especially carbohydrates, to energy. Therefore, many people reason that if they're tired, B-complex capsules will give them a boost of energy and improve their work performance. However, the amount of B-vitamin catalysts we need is directly related to the amount of carbohydrates burned. The B vitamins are contained in fresh whole-carbohydrate foods in optimal amounts, and taking extra won't provide any additional benefits. Double-blind scientific studies show no difference in work performance between those taking vitamins and those taking placebos. In fact, excessive amounts of nicotinic acid inhibit the ability of the heart muscle to use fatty acids as a fuel source. Supplements of the B complex of vitamins containing nicotinic acid should not be taken before strenuous activity.

The Pritikin diet contains a wide variety of unprocessed foods as grown and is rich in vitamins. Vitamin supplements not only are uncalled for, but are potentially hazardous to your health.

MINERALS

Recently, runners have become interested in mineral supplements, especially of the trace minerals known as electrolytes. These supplements have become quite popular now, and people are paying premium prices for fancy artificially flavored and colored powdered beverage mixes containing sugar, sodium, and potassium. However, only the *fluid* lost in perspiration needs to be replaced, and electrolyte supplements are unnecessary. Even with up to a four percent loss of body weight through sweating, mineral loss is small. Compared with other body fluids, sweat is hypotonic, which means the concentration of sodium, potassium, and other electrolytes in perspiration is more dilute than in the body tissues. In fact, it is the most dilute solution produced by the body. There will be some loss of minerals in prolonged sweating, but they are more highly concentrated in body tissues after dehydration. In addition, during exercise, glycogen in the liver and muscle cells frees up potassium to increase its concentration in the blood. Supplemental electrolytes could result in a disastrous imbalance.

Any potassium lost during exercise is easily replaced at the next meal if it is generous in unrefined foods. Lean, well-trained athletes have especially large potassium reserves because muscle cells contain more potassium than any other tissue. To reiterate: The main loss in sweat is water, and that is what needs to be replaced. If you drink water supplemented with even small amounts of sugar and electrolytes, it will take longer to pass through your stomach and into the tissues, where the fluid is needed. Plain water is the best thing to drink before, during, and after exercise, and it's important to do so on long runs, whether you feel thirsty or not, to meet your body's fluid needs. And remember that salting your food or taking salt tablets can dangerously increase your need for fluids.

It doesn't matter whether we are sedentary, active, or champion athletes. If we eat a variety of foods, primarily of plant origin, that have not been highly processed, we will not need or benefit from taking vitamin, mineral, or protein supplements or any other magic potion. In the next section, we will take a hard look at more of the myths held by both athletes and nonathletes.

3

The Great American Beer Controversy and Other Myths

Runners are especially sensitive to any information on ways to improve their performance. Some of them are always looking for a "magic potion" to give them an extra edge on their competition, and they eagerly scan nutrition publications for the advice of "experts."

Tom Bassler, M.D., has been featured widely in most running magazines and regularly writes letters to the editors of many medical journals. Bassler's popularity demonstrates the power of self-proclaimed nutrition experts. His opinions carry great weight because he has run marathons and is active in the AMJA (American Medical Joggers Association), an association of physicians who run. You can judge the wisdom of the following statements he has made:

> Beer is a good drink for the marathoner. It replaces the potassium you sweat out during a run which helps prevent heart attacks.

Beware! The carbonation and the bitterness of the beer make it taste good when you're hot and thirsty. However, it will not only make you feel hotter shortly after the first few quaffs, but it will greatly increase your chances of sustaining heat injury.

Your body will absorb the alcohol in beer quite rapidly, so that the sedative-hypnotic effects occur quickly. Some beer-drinking runners support their choice for fluid replacement on its potassium content. However, eight ounces of orange juice or a large banana has 8½ times the potassium of eight ounces of beer. You'll recall that there's no need to replenish trace minerals during competitive events. In fact, it can be harmful to do so. Vitally important, though, is that water be replaced. For that reason, beer is the last thing an athlete should drink, especially when performing on a hot day. Alcohol acts as a diuretic (stimulating urination) and causes dehydration. Drinking beer could cause death from heatstroke. Drinking two or more beers could put you to sleep forever.

Here is more evidence about the dangers of alcohol. Jay Bock, M.D., of the University of Florida, did a crossover study with 20 asymptomatic men, 26–65 years old. On one night, half had orange juice; the other half had orange juice with two ounces of vodka. Continuous monitoring while they were asleep demonstrated that the alcohol drinkers experienced 110 apneic events in which the breathing stopped for ten seconds or more, compared with only 20 events for those on orange juice. Apneic events are often the cause of death because they could initiate ventricular fibrillation, which leads to sudden death, even while you are asleep.

Don Jones, who refuses to take his megadoses of vitamin C, tore his Achilles.

The U.S. Air Force studied 286 officers (*JAMA*, 1970, *211:* 105) to see if there was a difference in the rate, severity, and duration of athletic injury sustained by those taking 1,000 mg of vitamin C a day compared with those taking a placebo. No difference was found.

No cases of death due to coronary atherosclerosis have been recorded in marathon finishers.

Years after evidence appeared in medical journals describing marathon runners' deaths from coronary events, Bassler continued to deny the correlation between running and coronary atherosclerosis in some deaths. (See Chapter 9 on runners' deaths.) Since the evidence is now overwhelming that runners *do* die of heart disease, Bassler has evolved the theory that runners' deaths are the result of "nutritional arrhythmia," citing nutritional reasons, especially a low-fat (ten percent) diet.

Some examples follow:

When I first saw the death certificate of Arne Richards, I knew it was wrong. . . . I knew that was another nutritional arrhythmia. . . . [Arne drank a lot of tea.] *Tea has a lot of phytates*—blocks absorption of metals (producing mineral deficiency). Arne just did not have the nutrients he needed to train in the hot Kansas climate.

Tea has *no* phytates.

For marathoners, the Pritikin diet or the "idealized Tarahumara diet" is dangerous because there isn't enough linoleic acid to protect cardiac function. Marathoners burn about 50 calories of linoleic acid for each mile beyond the 20-km (12-mile) mark. Any diet with only ten percent fat will have only five percent of the calories as linoleic acid . . . and remember that five percent of 2,000 calories is only 100 calories a day. . . . If anyone tried to run marathons regularly on the 80-10-10 Pritikin diet he should be dead or disabled in 18 months.

By this time, Bassler had shifted his position and conceded that marathoners do die suddenly—but from nutritional arrhythmia, because he claimed that on a 10-percent-fat diet there would be a deficiency of linoleic acid, an essential fatty acid. It is well known that runners require about 300 calories of fat each hour from their fat stores for energy. Perhaps Dr. Bassler thought that the 300 calories of fat required was linoleic acid, a fat eaten in small quantities but essential because the body can't make it.

By his reasoning, a runner would have to eat 300 calories of linoleic acid for every hour of running, or risk death. If a marathoner were to drink peanut oil, which Dr. Bassler recommends, he would have to drink 16 ounces or 1½ quarts for a ten-hour triathlon!

The point again is that the energy you derive from fat for running doesn't come from fat that you eat. It comes from your adipose tissue, where fat is stored after being metabolized from all three large nutrients—protein, carbohydrates, and fats.

The body makes all the fat you need from protein, carbohydrates, and fat, as present in ordinary foods, with one exception. Humans cannot make essential fatty acids. However, if you eat at least one percent of your total calories in essential fatty acids you will meet the body's requirement. The essential fatty acids are found primarily in whole grains—oats, whole wheat, brown rice, corn, barley, millet—and in lesser amounts in other plant foods (fruits, vegetables, and legumes).

Energy for muscular work comes primarily from glucose (carbohydrate) and fat. The fat you eat is not directly used for energy after it is digested and absorbed from the small intestine but goes to the adipose (fat) tissue in the form of triglycerides, which, you will recall, are composed of three fatty acids, referred to as FFA, or free fatty acids, plus glycerol. When the muscles call for fuel, the free fatty acids are released and provide about 50 percent of the calories used. A runner would probably use about 300 calories of FFA per hour.

Bassler's error was in stating that runners use 300 calories of *essential* fatty acids (EFA). In fact, the research to which Bassler referred stated specifically that runners use 300 calories of *free* fatty acids (FFA).

Bassler also stated that "During prolonged running, linoleic acid [an essential fatty acid] is specifically utilized as an energy substrate"—in other words, required for fuel, or energy, during running. Checking Bassler's sources indicates that he misread the information he used and thus reported it incorrectly. In fact, buring 300 calories of FFA presents no problem. The average athlete has 15 percent body fat—or at 150 pounds, 22 pounds of fat. Each pound can convert to FFA sufficient to run for eleven hours.

Even if it were true that runners needed much more linoleic acid, the Pritikin diet would still be the diet of choice, because it provides three to four times the amount you need. Medical studies establish that on a 10-percent-fat Pritikin-type diet, the adipose tissue has 60 percent more linoleic acid than on the 42-percent-fat American diet. This higher linoleic, or essential fatty acid, reserve, gives you greater protection against any possibility of essential fatty acid deficiency.

Another Bassler misreading of a medical study occurred with peanut butter. Bassler advocates peanut oil because it contains 25 percent linoleic acid. In order to get 300 calories of linoleic acid per hour to meet his recommendation for runners, you would have to eat 1,200 calories (⅓ pound) of peanut butter for every hour of running.

If we read carefully the medical study he quotes as his peanut butter justification (Smith, *Lancet* 1980, 1:534), we would learn the following:

> Peanut oil contains about 60 percent oleic acid (18:1) and 25 percent linoleic acid (18:2) and so theoretically it should be a "good" oil. . . . Extensive studies have now been reported . . . and in all the trials the most severe atherosclerotic lesions [narrowing or closure of the coronary arteries by cholesterol and fat deposits] in both aorta and coronary arteries were produced by peanut oil. . . . Serum cholesterol levels remained low on peanut oil.

There are at least 50 errors in Bassler's nutritional recommendations but he lets himself off the hook by saying, "You've got to make your own decision. After all, I might be wrong."

Subsequent to the publication in running magazines of Bassler's article on nutritional arrhythmia and other irresponsible reports on nutrition, the Community Nutrition Institute warned that "runners and other fitness enthusiasts who rely on the nation's major running magazines for diet advice are more likely to be confused than helped." The editor of *The Community Nutritionist,* Stephen Clapp, says running magazines do not provide sound, consistent advice on nutrition. In his article "Always Say Diet" (*The Community Nutritionist,* Nov./Dec. 1982), Clapp summarizes the current national dietary recommendations:

> 1. The National Academy of Sciences reports that the high amount of fat eaten in the American diet is a principal cause of breast, colon, and prostate cancer. Not only does the Academy advise the substantial reduction of all fats, but it cites evidence that polyunsaturated fats, such as are found in corn oil, vegetable margarines, safflower oil, sunflower-seed oil, and the like, increase the incidence of colon cancer more than the same amount of saturated fats, like butter or lard. Fats are out.
>
> 2. The American Heart Association has reconfirmed its position favoring a low-fat and low-cholesterol diet because of a "high correlation between the estimated level of fat (and cholesterol) in the diet and the severity of atherosclerosis."
>
> 3. The U.S. Dietary Guidelines and the Senate Nutrition Committee's *Dietary Goals* recommend cutting back on all fats, both saturated and polyunsaturated, and cholesterol.

Clapp continues: "There is nutritional expertise available to the editors of running magazines but they choose not to use it. If the running magazines were as irresponsible in medical matters as they are about nutrition, the readers would be offered cures by orgone therapy and phrenology."

"Readers," Clapp says, "*are* eager for sound nutrition information as part of their fitness programs. Reader surveys show that diet advice ranks with training tips among the most popular features. . . . The running magazines," he says, "should catch up with the times." He urges running magazines to hire nutrition editors who "should either be formally trained in nutrition or have the background and intelligence needed to separate sound advice from quackery."

4

What the Joggers Say

We're inundated with letters and stories from athletic people telling of their enthusiasm for the Pritikin diet. We hear from people who run three times a week for half an hour and from those who compete in marathons or triathlons, and we hear from children and from the elderly. We hear from women and from men. We hear from people who were sick when they started running, as well as from those who were healthy.

The following letter from Jill Kennedy of Glen Ellyn, Illinois, who is involved in running, bicycling, and other sports, is just one example:

> I've always eaten a high complex carbohydrate diet with maybe 20–30 percent fat—better than the average American—because that's what I liked, not because it was "good for me." I am 25 years old, athletic and extremely energetic. (My friends would say I am stating that mildly!) I became interested in your program through your articles in *Runner's World* magazine. The two things that attracted me were: (1) it seemed very similar to the diet I was eating, and (2) the people I admire most are endurance athletes

and many of these people, like the top finishers each year in the Ironman Triathlon and Rob de Castella, the world-champion marathoner, eat that way and believe it has helped improve their endurance and race times.

I bought all your books and became truly enthusiastic this past February. After reading your books I started looking at my diet more in terms of what was best for my overall health and kind of forgot the fitness aspect.

One of the many sports I do is run, and I've just gotten into racing 10Ks in the past year. My first race was in June 1983 and it was also my best race at 49:50. All my other race times have averaged around 51 minutes. Then in February 1984 I cut down to 10 percent fat and no sugar or salt in my diet. My first 10K of the year was two weeks ago and I beat my old record by over three minutes with a P. R. of 46:43! Wow! All of a sudden it hit me that this was the result of changing my diet!

Then, to top it off—I was in my first biathlon this past weekend which consisted of a 10K run and 30K bike race. I had decided to just run easy and finish, and not worry about any records. I finished the run in 44:42—another two minutes off my record of two weeks before! Incredible! I didn't even realize I was running so well. My training hasn't changed at all since last year—the only change I can notice is in my diet. I just had to write you and share my exciting news. Thanks for all the knowledge I've gained from your writings. P. S. I also have to tell you that even though this was my first biathlon, I came in the eighth woman of 76 women, finishing 176th in a field of 400 people!

Another vivid testimonial to the effectiveness of the program is the next letter from Wayne Jewell of Tujunga, California.

I have known of your work and have followed your progress since the early 1970s, when I was a photography student at Brooks Institute in Santa Barbara. I lived in a run-down apartment by the bird refuge. It was during this time that your patients overtook the bicycle paths along the East Beach and at the bird refuge.

A year or two later I saw you on "60 Minutes" with Mike Wallace, and I remarked "There's the guy with the old people who used to run by at the bird refuge."

It's ten years later now and you're part of my life every day. I've been an alcoholic for the last seven years, and last year my doctor told me that within ten years I would die of either liver failure or heart failure. At age 32 (last year) I had a cholesterol level over 300 and high blood pressure and early stages of liver failure.

Through the Employee Assistance Program at Anheuser-Busch, where I work, I was put in the care of a psychotherapist who specializes in the treatment of alcoholics. I've worked hard this past year, "slaying dragons" and "quieting voices" inside me. My mind, soul, and emotions were getting better but I was still overweight.

Two months ago we started a contest at Anheuser-Busch for overweight people called "Bubble-Buds." I decided it was time for me to let go of my alcohol, fat, and cholesterol. I entered the contest, determined that I was going to win, because I remembered Nathan Pritikin and his disciples at the bird refuge. . . .

Needless to say, I won the contest. In three months I've lost 40 pounds and have been able to increase my running to two miles four times a week. In March of 1985, I'm going to run a leg of the Jimmy Stewart American Heart Association Marathon in Griffith Park. Anheuser-Busch is a corporate sponsor each year, and we enter a team of five.

Thank you, "Coach," for saving my physical life. I not only look trimmer and slimmer, but look younger. . . . Is there any such thing as a Pritikin T-shirt? I'd be proud to wear one in my first 5K race.

Thanks again, Coach.

Three months after Mr. Jewell's September letter, he tells us his cholesterol level has come down from 350 to 237 mg/dl.

The following letter illustrates how much can be accomplished in as little as two weeks on the diet. Chris Summers of Los Angeles writes:

I am a 31-year-old woman, overweight, and just at the stage in my life where I was beginning to realize that fat and thirty is not a pleasure.

Approximately one month ago, I joined a health club and began working out three to four times a week with Nautilus equipment. Part of the program was a warm-up on a treadmill, and a few minutes on a "Life Cycle." Last month, I was considering myself very fortunate to do five minutes on either without feeling like I was going to pass out.

I have tried different diets, mostly stressing high protein, and usually wound up gaining weight. I work for two chiropractors, both of whom stress nutrition in their practice. I do dietary counseling, and make up menu plans. One doctor suggested I try a high carbohydrate diet. That afternoon found me at the bookstore to purchase *The Pritikin Promise*.

I have been on the diet for approximately two weeks, and I am delighted so far, and happy in the knowledge that things will only get better. Last night, at the health club, I did 30 minutes on the Life Cycle, and could have done 30 more. I have more endurance working out with weights; I no longer suffer with fluid retention. I wake up in the morning free from sausage fingers and under-eye puffiness, and a horrible taste in my mouth. My blood pressure is down to 110/70 from last month's 135/80. My pulse rate is slower. I have lost four pounds already, and I can see inches dropping, too.

I have energy all day long, I am much more mentally alert, and I feel wonderful. I no longer experience the little aches and pains that were always sending me to my bosses for a chiropractic adjustment. I used to wake up with stiff, painful knees and a stiff neck—but no more.

I am excited to see how I feel at the end of three months, three years . . . .

Thank you!

The three letters that follow are from young women who enjoy exercising with their husbands.

A 47-year-old woman from Vermont went from an arthritic cripple to a hiker and now takes dancing lessons and leads an active life with her husband.

I am writing to thank you for the incredible change your diet has made in my life. I am a 47-year-old woman who had polio as a small child, which left me with scoliosis (curvature of the spine). About 20 years ago, I started to develop arthritis in my spine, hip, and knee. I have been in all kinds of therapy with extensive drug therapy—all with only temporary results.

About four years ago, I decided to stop taking all drugs, including the vast quantities of aspirin. I tried in vain to live with the constant pain. Each winter in Vermont became more and more difficult. Last winter was the worst ever. I was on the verge of returning to drugs, when I happened to read an article in *House and Garden* about your diet.

I decided it was worth a try. Only four months later, fifteen pounds lighter and feeling twenty years younger, I found that all the stiffness in my back and leg had disappeared and about 80 percent of the pain was also gone. Every day I walk three miles to work. As you know, I live in Vermont, near the Green Mountains. On weekends, my husband and I try to take long hikes of possibly five to seven miles. I am taking a dance class twice a week. All of this from someone whose favorite expression used to be "my idea of exercise is getting up in the morning!" I can't believe the energy I have, and neither can my husband.

Another interesting thing happened. My premenstrual symptoms, which were becoming more intense as I approached menopause, have all but disappeared. No more depression, cramping, and headaches. Fantastic! Again, thank you for your diet. Thank you for giving me a new life to live.

Thirty-nine-year-old Robert Christensen of West Babylon, New York, ran faster after going on the diet and improved in competitive events. His 31-year-old wife tells their story:

This is the first diet I have ever been on that I could stay on and not have a weak and faint feeling, and on which I could lose weight so fast. I lost seven pounds in three weeks, and my husband lost approximately 15 pounds in one month. My husband is a runner and runs about 60 miles a week.

Since he started the diet, he runs much faster and has placed among the top three in his age group in many races. We love the diet and have never felt better. Before reading your book, my husband would consume a pound of butter or margarine in less than a week, with approximately 21 eggs per week, besides drinking alcohol. I can't tell you what a wonderful change your diet has made in our lives. Thank you.

The Kochers of Gardnerville, Nevada, are husband and wife marathoners. Thirty-five-year-old Patricia wrote to tell us of the benefits she and her husband derived from the diet.

My husband and I are both runners, and I have been running almost five years. I am 35 years old, and five feet tall, so when I weighed 115 pounds, before starting your diet, I was trying to lose weight. Once I went on your diet, I had no problem getting the weight off and am at my present weight of 101 pounds.

I noticed a big difference in performance after going on your diet. My average running mile used to be 9:45; now at a racing speed, up to half a marathon, I do a 7:50 mile. In winter, we usually do 20–25 miles per week. Ordinarily, in other seasons, we average 33 miles per week, unless we are training for a marathon.

If I go off the diet for more than one meal, I can tell the difference not only in energy but mood changes. We have both been acutely aware that even a moderate change in our habits has affected our daily feeling of well-being as well as performance.

Brothers Bill and Frank Beddor and Frank's sons, Steve and David, are a family of runners. Bill, age 56, ran his first marathon after his 50th birthday. Eager to test his endurance, he entered the 100-mile Western States Endurance Run in June 1979. This race involves desert, mountains, snow, heat, and pain. After 64 miles, he had to give up, exhausted in body and mind.

In January of 1980, Bill started the Pritikin Program; and with his new energy, he entered the June 1980 Endurance Run. This time he finished the 100 miles in 29 hours.

But 1982 was Bill's banner year:

- June, 1982: Western States 100-Mile Race—22:55.
- October, 1982: Ironman Triathlon—third in his age group, 13:48.

Bill's new goals:

- 100-mile run—less than 20 hours.
- Ironman Triathlon—less than 12 hours.
- Diet—100 percent Pritikin for the rest of his life.

Frank, inspired by Bill's new energy, started the Pritikin Program in September 1980 and persuaded his sons, Steve and David, to go on the diet. Although neither father nor sons put enough time into their training, in June 1981, Steve, 20, ran his first marathon with his father and finished.

October 10, 1982, the *Minneapolis Tribune* ran this story: "Beddors win 50-miler. Frank Beddor, Jr., 58, and son David, 20, finished first in the father-son division at last weekend's Michigan 50-Mile Ultramarathon. Frank was the oldest finisher, David the youngest."

5

High Performance on the Pritikin Diet

Even world-class endurance athletes thrive on the Pritikin diet. They follow the same diet program as active ten-year-olds, fifty-year-olds who have just started a walking program, and ninety-year-olds who simply want to feel better. Everyone benefits and can function at his or her optimal level physically and mentally on this nutritional program. Remember, the best made car in the world will never perform at its maximum on low quality fuel, and you will never reach your potential on the nutritionally poor high-fat diet eaten by most Americans.

The Hawaii Ironman Triathlon is a grueling annual event consisting of a 2.4-mile ocean swim, 112-mile bicycle race, and a 26.2-mile marathon run. For six weeks prior to the 1982 Ironman, Dave Scott, Scott Tinley, and Scott Molina were monitored as they trained on the Pritikin diet. In Hawaii, a special Pritikin kitchen was set up for their meals. On the day of the '82 Hawaii Triathlon, the heat was almost unbearable, and the black asphalt road reached temperatures up to 115°F.

On October 9, 1982, 850 entrants started the Hawaii Iron-man Triathlon. The winners:

PLACE	RUNNER	AGE	TIME
First	Dave Scott	28	9:08:23*
Second	Scott Tinley	25	9:28:28
Third	Jeff Tinley	22	9:36:53
	(Scott's brother)		
Fourth	Scott Molina	22	9:40:23

To Scott Molina, his fourth place finish was a great victory. In the 1981 contest he had been running in second place when exhaustion and dehydration forced him out less than ten miles from the finish. This time, he was a strong finisher.

Dave Scott had won the 1980 triathlon in 9:24, but in February 1982 he finished 17 minutes behind Scott Tinley's world record time of 9:10. To regain first place in October 1982 was a great satisfaction, but to do it with a new record time of 9:08:23, 16 minutes faster than his best time, made it even sweeter. He also won each individual event.

Dave had been following his own version of the Pritikin diet for several years and preparing his own food. He still does. He's been on the diet for nine years now. He cooks up two pounds of brown rice and leaves it on the stove, and eats it all through the day, along with yogurt, vegetables, and up to 20 pieces of fruit per day.

This gives him all the calories he needs for those eight-hour training days, and replenishes the glycogen stores in his muscles for the next day. An 80 percent carbohydrate diet means continuous carbohydrate loading, and no one uses up more glycogen than Dave Scott, the best endurance athlete in the world.

After the 1982 Triathlon, Dave said: "Over the past seven

---

* Since the Hawaii Triathlon started in 1978, only three other athletes have broken the ten-hour total time for the triple event.

years I have been following a strict but enjoyable diet—I do enjoy eating—of approximately ten percent of my total calories in fat, fifteen percent in protein, and 75 percent in complex carbohydrates. This diet has undoubtedly contributed to my athletic performance in triathlons over the last five years. The total reduction of fat and cholesterol, with an increase in muscle and liver glycogen through a higher carbohydrate diet has enabled me to train for five to eight hours daily and to compete at a world-class level.''

In the 1983 Ironman, once again, Dave Scott came in first and Scott Tinley came in second. In October 1984, Dave finished in 8 hours, 54 minutes and 20 seconds, shattering his own course record by more than ten minutes and beating the runner-up by 24 minutes. Second place? Scott Tinley.

Compare Dave with another triathlon entrant, age 22, 6 feet, 151 pounds, who finished in 14½ hours. His diet? Red meat, most days; eggs, whole milk. As he admits, he was one typical American when it came to his dietary habits.

In October 1982, the 850 participants of the Ironman Triathlon were polled as to their food habits and preferred diet. Over 50 percent answered the questionnaire. Half of the athletes selected the Pritikin diet as their number-one choice. In reviewing their intake of fats and cholesterol, I could see they had a good understanding of the guidelines of the Pritikin diet. As athletes continue to push for higher levels of endurance I believe more of them will try to adopt this high performance diet.

TENNIS ANYONE?

Martina Navratilova, the world's number-one-seeded tennis player—over two million dollars in earnings in 1984—has come back to the top in women's tennis after a few years of not playing as well as she wanted to. Now even Chris Evert Lloyd can barely keep up with her. Ms. Navratilova started a new diet in 1982. "No fats, no oils, no butter, no red meats, no sugar," she explains. "Plenty of vegetables and carbohydrates."

That means, she said, eating a lot of unadorned pasta, potatoes, and bread, which she admitted was not easy at first for someone who used to like things "swimming in butter."

After several months on the diet, she said, "I feel stronger." And in world-class competition, you need all the strength and endurance you can get.

RUNNERS: WORLD CLASS!

Robert de Castella, marathoner.

In three years, Robert had gone from a promising young runner to, as Ron Clarke, a former world champion runner, described it, the winner of the greatest marathon yet run—the 1982 Commonwealth Games in Brisbane, Australia.

In 1981 he won the Japanese Fukuoka out-and-back marathon in 2:08:18, five seconds longer than Alberto Salazar's world record for the one-way course New York marathon. Although the distance is the same, there is a difference in degree of difficulty. The one-way course of 26 miles in the New York marathon was fast because the runners were given a little extra boost from a favorable wind. In an out-and-back course, you run the 13-mile mark, then turn back to the starting point. In this way, any favoring winds or downhill advantages are averaged.

Robert set a world record for an out-and-back marathon and is setting his sights on U.S. marathons. In 1982 he beat Bill Rodgers and Frank Shorter, among other great runners. On April 9, 1983, Robert raced Alberto Salazar in a world-class marathon in Holland. It was their first race. Robert won first place, and Alberto came in fifth. Alberto said he had kept up with Robert for the first 22 miles and that Robert had then taken off like a rocket. A convincing demonstration of the high-carbohydrate diet's effect on endurance. Because marathons are so stressful, Robert has run only nine since he started, ten years ago. Unlike many other long-distance runners, he has had an almost injury-free record, and he recovers quickly from minor injuries.

In 1976 Robert's diet changed radically. His father, Rolet, an ex-Army man, had always been very fit and disciplined about his health. He had run for years. Suddenly, in 1974, he had a stroke, and nine months later, a heart attack that completely disabled him.

Rolet read an interview with me in *Runner's World* in 1976 describing my success using diet to restore heart disease victims to normal function. Rolet contacted me, and I sent him the diet program. Robert describes his father's improvement:

> Dad was always very fit and ran a lot, but when he had his heart attack, he could hardly get out of bed to walk upstairs without bad angina for almost a year. Then he put himself on a very stringent nonfat, nonsalt diet with mainly complex carbohydrates, such as potatoes, pumpkins, and other vegetables, cereals and grains. Since then, he's run sixteen marathons, the most recent when he ran three hours and twelve minutes, a very good run for a man of 58. Now he gets no angina at all.

Robert adopted his father's diet in 1977—nonfat, nonsalt, with no meat, cheese or eggs, and is not concerned about a heart attack, even if he may have a hereditary tendency. "I think my diet and running will protect me from a heart attack," he says.

This father and son have demonstrated quite clearly that the magic for endurance is simply proper nutrition.

WORLD-RECORD RUNNER (65–69 AGE GROUP)

Jack Stevens, now 68, holds world records for 400, 800, and 1,600 meters.

	AGE	METERS	TIME	METERS	TIME
1974	58	800	2:21:3 (record)	1,600	5:11
Jan 82	65	800	2:24:3 (record)		
April 10, 1982			Started Pritikin Diet		
May 82	65	800	2:22:9 (record)		
Aug 82	65	800	2:20:5 (record)		
Nov 82	65			1,600	4:50:6 (record)

JACK STEVENS AT 65 HAS MADE AN ASTONISHING DISCOVERY
(An interview condensed from *Prime Time,* December, 1982, Melbourne, Australia)

His physical prowess is improving. He recently ran 800 meters faster than he did seven years ago, breaking his own world record in the process. Jack's wife is a remarkable athlete as well, and though she started discus and javelin only five years ago when she was 60, she is already an American/Australian champion. Diet, they say, is the magic key to their feats. In April 1982 they decided to try the diet devised by U.S. scientist Nathan Pritikin. It is a low fat, low cholesterol, high carbohydrate eating pattern. Pritikin claims that by sticking to his diet people find new energy and health in old age and in fact at any age.

This diet for Jack and Maisie is now a way of life. Jack was a top athlete in the late 1950s, and at 65, although he had slowed a little he still set a new world record for the 800 meters in the 65–69 age group, 2:24:3.

Half a year later, after starting the new diet, he broke his own world record by a stunning four seconds, 2:20:5 in the Philadelphia National Masters Sports Festival. His fellow athletes were awestruck. He said the only thing he had done differently was switch to the Pritikin diet.

Maisie's story is similar. She took up the discus and javelin five years ago after being on angina tablets for ten years, because she was bored just watching her husband compete. Since starting the Pritikin diet, she gradually reduced the number of tablets for her angina, and now she takes none at all. Her arthritis is gone too, and she has lost 17 pounds. "It's the healthiest I have been in years," she said. "With angina, I couldn't walk up even a slight hill without being totally knocked out by it." This year she is an Australian/American champion in both the discus and the javelin.

Jack writes his own story:

For the past 11 years, I have been competing in Veteran (Masters) athletics, running mainly the 400- and 800-meter races. I turned 65 years old on November 23, 1981. The next 12 months changed my life.

December 11, 1981, I had a stress treadmill test, and the heart specialist said that my systolic blood pressure was too high—whether I was on the treadmill or not—and to come back for treatment.

January 23, 1982, I ran the 800 meters in 2:24:5, a new world's record. The old one was 2:25:3, held by Frank Finger, U.S.A. One week later, I ran the 400 meters in 62.17. This bettered slightly the world record also held by Frank Finger, U.S.A. Having retired on my 65th birthday, I decided to change my diet around that time by a large increase in the number of eggs I consumed and also a big intake in cream. But I didn't feel well after that, and I went to my physician again, and he checked me out and found my blood pressure much too high.

April 8, 1982, I decided to go back to the heart specialist. He told me that something must be done with my blood pressure and tried to figure out what drugs I would have to take, and he would try to choose the ones least likely to affect my running.

April 10, 1982, I found your book *The Pritikin Program for Diet and Exercise.* We were almost immediately on your diet.

April 29, 1982, I saw the heart specialist, and that was only two weeks after I started your diet, and he said my blood pressure was much better, and he would postpone ordering the medication. I told him about my diet change, but he was not impressed. He said I should be having a "balanced" diet, including some meat and eggs. I told him that I would go by the way I feel. I was due to race in Fiji in May of 1982, and he made another appointment to see me after Fiji.

May 13, 1982, in Fiji, I ran a good 800-meter race in 2:22:9, which shaved 1.6 seconds off my previous record. At about the same time, I was finding that in my training I was able to do things that I could not manage for several years before that. The only thing different was the diet change.

June 3, 1982, I saw the heart specialist again. He found my blood pressure now normal. But he isn't convinced that it is due to the Pritikin diet, like I am. He says, "Well, it's just psychological, just due to a diet change." It's hard to convince the doctors.

August, 1982, we traveled to America to compete first in Wichita, Kansas, and a week later in Philadelphia where I broke records again, the fastest times I have been able to achieve in the last seven years. I feel I owe it to the diet. I no longer "die" during the second half of the race, and the improvement was quite noticeable even after being on the diet a little more than a month.

Now regarding my wife, Maisie, who turned 65 in 1982. She has been in the doctor's hands for angina for the last 15 years. She has had to seek treatment earlier this year for what was diagnosed as a hiatus hernia. She has suffered with arthritis in the knee joints for some years, even though she has been competing in discus and javelin for the last two and a half to three years. On her change to the Pritikin system, her weight went from 133 down to 112, and her knees are now practically free of any discomfort and she joins me in many running training sessions. Her hiatus hernia is nonexistent and, over a period of almost six weeks, she gradually cut down her angina tablets and in a month after that she was without medication of any kind.

Maisie and I are both feeling the best we have felt in years. After 43 years of marriage, we claim to be the happiest couple in the world and we agree that the Pritikin Program has had a lot to do with it.

IT'S NEVER TOO LATE TO START!

Noel Johnson improves with age.

AGE
69 Recommended for nursing home; denied life insurance
70 Drastically changed diet to Pritikin guidelines
71 Ran a 6:27 mile
73 Pike's Peak Marathon
80 New York Marathon
82 New York Marathon
83 New York Marathon

At 70 years old, despite medical advice not to exercise, Noel began his own rehab program of diet and exercise. He changed his diet drastically: no meat, cheese, eggs, butter, margarine, or oils; essentially a plant food diet with a small amount of animal protein—fish once or twice a week.

Noel wrote me, "I know that your way of life as stated in your book, free from so many damaging oils, has helped me to obtain the physical condition I have at 83."

Eula Weaver, almost 91 years old at her last competition. Record holder for 800 meters (85–89 years old) and 1,500 meters (85–89 years old and 90–94 years old) at Senior Olympics event, 1974 to 1979.

Five feet three inches tall, Eula had weighed 100 pounds for the last 40 years. She developed heart disease with angina at 67, and at 75 years old she was hospitalized with a severe heart attack. At 81, she had congestive heart failure, angina, hypertension, severe arthritis, and claudication (not enough blood flow to the legs). She could walk no more than 100 feet. Circulation to her hands was so bad that she had to wear gloves in the summertime.

She started the Pritikin diet when she was 81 years old, and in a year was off all medication, had lost her symptoms, and could walk a mile. At the age of 85½, she entered the Senior

Olympics, ran the 800 and 1,500 meters, and won two gold medals. She ran these races for six consecutive years and won 12 gold medals.

It's never too late to start.

IN A CLASS BY THEMSELVES

- Monroe Rosenthal, M.D.   Marathon: 2:45; Ironman Triathlon: 12:08
- John Scheff, M.D.   Marathon: 3:00; Ironman Triathlon: 11:36.

Dr. Rosenthal writes:

As a doctor in Internal Medicine, specializing in diabetes, I was fascinated by your complete reversal of dietary recommendations for diabetics. From the 50 years of low carbohydrate, high fat diets, now studies were demonstrating superior results with high carbohydrate, low fat diets.

In late 1979 I read your book *The Pritikin Program for Diet and Exercise.* It made sense to me, especially after I read the chapter for health professionals documenting the scientific rationale for diabetics.

In February 1980 not only did I start your diet, but set up a metabolic ward in my hospital for my patients. Dramatic results were achieved with diabetes, hypertension, and heart disease.

My own performance was improving on the diet. The best marathon time before the diet was 2:59, but after four months on your diet, I ran a 2:45, my best time ever, and I qualified for the Boston Marathon, which required a 2:50 or faster time.

After three Boston Marathons, I turned to the ultimate contest, the Ironman World Triathlon in Hawaii. In the February 1982 Triathlon I was pleased with my 12:42, coming in 175th out of 650 entrants. What surprised me in my close association with the other triathletes and especially the top finishers, was that most of them were generally following the guidelines of the Pritikin diet.

To bring attention that your diet, although originally for sick people, was indeed the best for overall fitness in endurance athletes, I contacted you in February 1982 to do a study on triathletes training on your diet. Some 850 contestants entered the October 1982 race, and the six you sponsored won the first, second, and fourth places.

Another physician, John Scheff, and I were two of the six you sponsored. My October time was 12:08, 34 minutes faster than February. John had run marathons for a few years and did the February 1982 triathlon in 13:06. He went on your diet three or four months before the October event, and made a remarkable improvement in his time—from 13:06 to 11:36, one and a half hours less.

The consensus of the group was that the diet was significant in their improvements in time.

I continue to use your diet with my patients and am constantly in wonder of such a simple natural approach proving so effective.

- **Ed Wehan,** age 39. Marathon: 2:37; 50-mile: 5:53; 100-mile Western States: 18:48. Ed writes:

During college, I played competitive tennis on a diet of red meat and French fries. My roommate's father gave him a side of beef every semester, which we devoured. I sure wasn't born to a Pritikin diet. Around 1971, in my late twenties, I weighed too much, and started to run to gain conditioning. After a one-and-a-half-mile run, I would go home for a couple of Big Macs and fries which made it difficult for me to lose weight.

After considerable reading, I decided to cut back on simple carbos, fats, and oils. Weight started dropping off, and I was feeling better and was able to increase my running distance.

In 1976 I read your first book, and was surprised that most of my new food habits were your recommendations. I was about two-thirds on your diet and was ready for my first marathon. It was a nervous experience for me, but I finished in 3:30. The next year, I changed my diet in earnest and by 1978 was a strict follower.

In 1979, I ran the 100-mile Western States and finished seventh with an 18:48, and I now have run this race three times. Over 350 entrants were in the American River 50-miler, and I finished fourth in 5:53.

As far as marathons, I now run a 2:37, and two marathons were only two weeks apart. I seem to have very rapid recovery. Even my 10K is fast, 33:30.

I attribute my endurance to my diet. I train minimally, compared to most, and still perform well. As we age, I believe our diets can influence performance more than at a younger age. My company does fitness testing, and many of the older runners I test tend toward your type of diet. Although I'm 39, I look for my fastest times in the next 15 years.

SUPERMEN—THEIR NEXT EVENT

ultra-triathlon:　　{ 20-mile swim
48 to 60 hours,　　200-mile bicycle race
continuous-nonstop　　100-mile run

- Allan Korolowicz, age 29
- Craig Chambers, age 34

These runners are planning the ultimate triathlon, and if they pull it off, they will have duplicated the 200-mile-run endurance of the Tarahumara.

Allan, who is one of the top ultramarathoners in the world, recently did a 100-mile run across Death Valley, in 115–119°F air temperatures, with the roads reaching 180–190°F.

Craig was to run 50 miles to pace Allan, but ran 80 miles instead. Craig's development as a superendurance athlete is interesting to follow.

He started running in 1974, eating the typical high-fat American diet. As his distance increased, he started to eat more carbohydrates; then by 1978, he gave up fish, fowl, and meat and became a lacto-ovo-vegetarian. He had information on the

Pritikin diet and gradually began shifting away from the dairy products.

In April 1978 Craig ran his first marathon. The 26-mile distance inspired him to longer training runs, and by July of 1978, he was running 20 miles most days. A 50-mile race became a reality in September of 1978, and his best time is 6:07.

The next big challenge was the Western States 100-mile race. It's a wild run through desert, snow, mountains, etc., but he has run it three times, in 1980, 1981, and 1982, with a best time of 21:14.

By 1980, Craig felt stronger without the dairy products, and for his animal protein, ate a few eggs each week. His diet now was 10 percent fat and about 75–80 percent carbohydrates, following the Pritikin guidelines.

He felt so strong in 1981 that he raised his training runs to at least 24 miles a day, seven days a week, and over the past two years has run more than 17,000 miles—two-thirds around the world, or seven coast-to-coast runs. His greatest mileage week totaled 242 miles, or about 35 miles a day.

With this kind of training, he couldn't resist the Ironman Triathlon in 1981, and did it in 12:27. Now, after 30 marathons, with a best time of 2:47, he's aiming for the impossible, the ultratriathlon.

- Marathon a day (7 days a week) for 700 + continuous days
- 1981–82: 24 + miles of running daily without missing a day = 17,520 miles
- Marathon: 2:47
- 50-mile: 6:07
- Ironman Triathlon: 12:27
- Western States 100-mile: 21:14

And this is just the beginning for Craig "Superman" Chambers!

People aged 20 to 83 years, selected from the case histories, who were or became marathon (or more) runners while following the Pritikin guidelines for at least a year:

YEARS ON DIET	NAME	AGE	MARA-THON TIME	OTHER EVENTS
6	Irwin Baker	54	3:33	42-mile, 8:00
4	John Becker	42	2:57	
3	Bill Beddor	56	3:14	100-mile, 22:55; Ironman Triathlon, 13:48
3	David Beddor	20	4:00	50-mile winner
3	Frank Beddor	58	4:00	50-mile winner
3	Steve Beddor	21	4:00	
3	Irwin Berman	55	4:42	
3	Lloyd Brodniak	38	2:49	
3	Craig Chambers	34	2:47	50-mile, 6:07; 100-mile, 21:14; Ironman Triathlon, 12:27
6	Robert de Castella	25	2:08:18	Winner of 4/9/83 Rotterdam, Holland, Marathon, defeating Alberto Salazar
7	Rolet de Castella	59	2:58	
10	Noel Johnson	83	4:50	
2	Nick Karem	39	3:45	
3	Mr.&Mrs.Kocher	40, 35	4:00	
3	Allan Korolowicz	29		100-mile
2	Ridge La Mar	34	3:30	
1	Scott Molina	22	2:24	Ironman Triathlon. 9:40
5	Roger Nichols	35	3:00	
4	Hilda Richardson	67	6:10	
3	Debbie Robison	28	5:00	

YEARS ON DIET	NAME	AGE	MARA- THON TIME	OTHER EVENTS
3	Grace Robison	47	5:00	
3	Monroe Rosenthal	35	2:45	Ironman Triathlon, 12:08
2	R. T. Ryan	47	3:15	
1	John Scheff	30	3:00	Ironman Triathlon, 11:36
9	David Scott	30	sub 3:00	Ironman Triathlon, 8:54
3	Gina Serafin	44	5:03	
3	Tony Serafin	21	3:58	
2,000	Tarahumara Indians			200 miles, 48:00
6	Ed Wehan	39	2:37	50-mile, 5:53; 100-mile, 18:48

As you know, the Pritikin diet is based on the diet of the Tarahumaras in northern Mexico and 25 other native populations where the degenerative diseases (heart disease, cancer, etc.) are unknown. They have thrived on it for 2,000 years. How does their diet affect their endurance?

• They can carry loads of up to 80 percent of their weight 110 miles in 70 hours.
• They can run 500 miles in five days to deliver a letter (faster than the postal service).
• Six-year-olds kick a wooden ball the size of an orange six miles in 70 to 80 minutes. Adult men kick the ball 90 to 180 miles in 24 to 48 hours.
• A 43-year-old man has kicked the ball 36 miles in six hours, with postrace heart rate of 102.
• They hunt deer by running them into exhaustion in 24 to 48 hours.
• Whole families walk 180 miles to visit friends.

Women also have a kickball game, but because they're busy with food preparation and raising children, they run for *only* 50 miles!

By now you can see how thoroughly nutritious and safe the Pritikin diet is, even for people who tax their bodies to the limit. If you have any lingering doubts as to whether it's wise to forego high-fat-and-protein diets, the following chapter should put your mind to rest.

6

Run and Die on the American Diet

About six months before his death this year, Jim Fixx phoned me and criticized the chapter "Run and Die on the American Diet" in *The Pritikin Promise*. In that chapter, I documented my thesis that running is not protective against heart disease. I said that many runners on the average American diet have died and will continue to drop dead during or shortly after long-distance events or training sessions. Jim thought the chapter was hysterical in tone and would frighten a lot of runners. I told him that was my intention. I hoped it would frighten them into changing their diet. I explained that I think it is better to be hysterical before someone dies than after. Too many men, I told Jim, had already died because they believed that anyone who could run a marathon in under four hours and who was a nonsmoker had absolute immunity from having a heart attack.

Running can't offer this protection, and here's why. When you run, your heart needs more oxygen. To put a slight stress on your heart causes healthful adaptive changes to take place, and that's why aerobic exercise is good for you. However, if your diet is similar to that eaten by most Americans, it's high in fat and cholesterol which causes thickening and narrowing of the blood vessels supplying oxygen to the heart. When this occurs, strenuous exercise can cause an oxygen deficit so great that the heart goes into a fatal arrhythmia.

My copy of Jim's latest best-selling book, *Jim Fixx's Second Book of Running,* is inscribed with thanks for my help. Although Jim had used me as a source of information on many aspects of health, he failed to be convinced that a diet of 10 percent fat and 100 milligrams or less cholesterol a day was better than the American Heart Association (AHA) diet that limits fat to 30 percent and cholesterol to 300 milligrams daily. The most recent study of the AHA diet, the MRFIT seven-year, 12,000-man, $115,000,000 trial, demonstrated no difference in the incidence of heart disease or in the number of total deaths between those on the AHA diet and those on the average American diet.

When Jim said his doctor had told him his cholesterol level was normal, I explained that so-called "normal" refers to average American levels which are much higher than they should be. Most people, like Jim, don't know what their cholesterol level should be. Truly normal cholesterol levels are 100 plus your age, but not over 150–160. Jim's last reported cholesterol level was 253.

The large and famous Framingham study showed way back in 1958 that as your serum cholesterol increases, so does your risk of developing heart disease. The recent Chicago Heart Association study showed that deaths due to heart disease increase in the same degree of magnitude as incidence with rises in serum cholesterol. The findings of both groups of researchers are summarized in the following chart:

CHOLESTEROL SHOULD BE LESS THAN 160 mg/dl

CHOLESTEROL LEVEL mg/dl	Relative Risk of:	
	Developing Heart Disease	Dying of Heart Disease
	FRAMINGHAM STUDY*	CHICAGO HEART ASSOC.†
140–159	(114–193) 1	1
160–179		4.5
195–218	5.3	6.3
219–240	6.7	7.5
241–268	12.4	8.5
268 +	15.3	16.5

Lancet, Aug. 1982   † *Medical World News,* April 1983

These figures were published a year before Jim's death. Jim's "normal" cholesterol level of 253 gave him eight times more risk than if his cholesterol had been less than 150. This information could have saved Jim's life and could save yours, too.

Another marathoner whose sport did not protect him from dying of heart disease was Jacques Bussereau. Jacques died at the age of 48 while running the 1984 New York marathon. He did not have a history of heart disease and had run in four previous marathons. The event took place on an exceptionally hot and humid October day, but Dr. Andres Rodriquez, the medical director of the race, minimized the effect of the temperature, saying that heat causes exhaustion but does not cause sudden death. As with Jim Fixx, occlusive artery disease was found on autopsy.

Too many runners think diet doesn't make any difference and that they burn up cholesterol by running. This isn't true. Unlike fat, cholesterol cannot be burned for energy, and can only be excreted at a slow and fixed rate through the intestinal tract. If more is consumed than can be eliminated, the stores gradually accumulate, producing artery closure. Running or other forms of exercise will help your body rid itself of excess fat, but it won't do a thing for preventing artery closure from cholesterol buildup. Many runners pay with their lives for this misconception.

Another myth in vogue is that there is a good kind of cholesterol that protects against heart disease. Sometimes your blood test will give you not only the total amount of cholesterol in 100 milliliters of your blood but a few of the cholesterol fractions as well, one of which is your HDL cholesterol. If the HDL level is high, some people believe it will protect you from having a heart attack even though your total blood cholesterol is also high.

HDL cholesterol can be raised both by healthy lifestyle habits such as exercise or by unhealthy practices such as alcohol consumption. Regardless of the reason for a high level of HDL cholesterol, it won't protect you from heart disease. The average level is 31–60 milligrams per deciliter; Jim Fixx's was 87. Alcohol was probably responsible for the above-average level, since even the most sustained vigorous exercise can raise it only to about 60. He was told by the person administering the test that a total cholesterol level as high as his (above 250) was common among athletes because of their high level of HDL cholesterol, and that it was nothing to worry about. The belief that he was protected by his high HDL cost Jim his life.

Don't be like Jim and depend on running alone, or on a high HDL cholesterol reading. If you don't watch your diet, there is no protection.

Runners and nonrunners alike are misled by another fallacy as well—that if they have normal electrocardiograms, their hearts are not in danger. Most American men over the age of 40 have blockage in their coronary arteries that may not show up in treadmill testing or prevent them from running marathons. It is the blockage in the three pencil-slim coronary arteries that nourish the heart that produces fatal heart attacks. In a National Institutes of Health study of five runners who died while running, pathologists B. F. Waller and W. C. Roberts found all five to have been free of electrocardiographic or other evidence of heart disease before they started running. The lowest cholesterol level of the runners, however, was 228 mg/dl.

A third common misconception is the fatalistic belief that family history or genes will predetermine whether or not you will succumb to a heart attack. Practically all of us have a family history of heart disease because of acquired—not inherited—eating habits. Everyone on the typical American diet has a risk factor for heart disease. Only one in 500 have a hereditary risk factor for heart disease, and Jim Fixx was not one of those people. If he had changed his diet, he could have continued to run safely, or if he was reluctant to make dietary changes, he should have stopped running.

Compare Jim Fixx and Jacques Bussereau with the Australian marathoner, Rolet de Castella, whose son Robert is one of the world's greatest marathoners (see Chapter 5). Jim died at age 52 while running, and Rolet had a stroke at age 52 while running. During Rolet's recuperation, he suffered a heart attack and was completely disabled with angina (chest pains) for a year. He went on the Pritikin diet (10 percent fat, under 100 milligrams cholesterol daily) and his angina quickly lessened and disappeared as his circulation improved. He cautiously resumed running and in two years ran his first marathon. Before his heart attack, he was only a five-mile-a-day runner. He is now 60 and has run about 20 marathons in as short a time as three hours, a speed men half his age would be proud to do. His case proves that while running does not prevent heart disease, proper diet, even after a heart attack, can return you to an active, vigorous life, even that of a marathon runner.

Rolet's son, Robert, went on the Pritikin diet in 1977. In 1981 he won the Fukuoka Marathon in Japan in 2:08:18, five seconds slower than Alberto Salazar's world record for the

New York City Marathon. In 1982 he was the winner of the . Commonwealth Games event in Brisbane, Australia; and in 1983 he beat Salazar in the Rotterdam Marathon and came in first in the Helsinki World Championship. It's obvious to Robert that the Pritikin diet is doing great things for his endurance and performance. And he's not worried that he might have a family tendency toward heart disease, because he's convinced that his low-fat diet will protect him from having a heart attack.

Goodloe Byron, U.S. Congressman from Maryland, is another runner who thought his sport alone would provide adequate protection against his premature demise from heart disease. Byron had read extensively about health and running, and was intrigued by Dr. Tom Bassler's flat statement that anyone who runs a marathon in under four hours and is a nonsmoker has absolute immunity from heart disease. How wrong he was!

At the age of 49, Byron had run six Boston Marathons, with a best time of 3:28:40, and had finished a 50-miler. He was 5 feet 7 inches tall and weighed 130 pounds, had run almost every day for several years for at least half an hour, and had not smoked for 25 years. Then why, toward the end of an easy 15-mile training run, did he drop dead? Because he was so strongly influenced by the belief in the immunity of marathon runners to heart disease, he ignored his physician's warnings about his gradually closing coronary arteries, as shown in successive treadmill tests in 1974 to 1978. Dr. Robert Flynn, Byron's personal physician, said the last test, in January 1978, indicated severe abnormality and was positive for heart disease. "I advised him to stop running completely until further tests could be done with Dr. Sam Fox (head of the Cardiology Exercise Project of Georgetown University)."

Byron continued to run, and though he made four appointments with Dr. Fox in the next ten months, he canceled them because of his congressional work load. His cholesterol level in 1974 was 305 mg/dl, and in 1978, the year of his death, had

declined to 228 mg/dl. A safe cholesterol level would have
been below 160 mg/dl.

But Byron ignored his diet and his doctors. He believed that
running made him immune to heart disease. He died of heart
disease on October 12, 1978.

Dr. Manuel G. Jimenez, who did the autopsy, said the coronary arteries were filled with cholesterol, "extensive and dif-
fuse, involving both coronary arteries and main branches. The
coronaries were narrowed to only pinprick openings. Congressman Byron's coronary arteries were worse than most
I've autopsied."

After receiving the autopsy report, Dr. Bassler said the
death had not been caused by heart disease. "He probably
wasn't eating one of the six foods that [Bassler recommends]
marathoners eat: yeast, yogurt, peanuts, beer, wheat germ
and vitamin C."

Dr. Jimenez politely commented that Bassler's conclusions
were *not* supported by the evidence: ". . . for me, it was
plainly coronary insufficiency due to atherosclerosis."

The information about Byron's untimely death comes from
a study of sudden death in marathon runners on the regular
American diet that was conducted by B. F. Waller and W. C.
Roberts, pathologists at the National Institutes of Health. In
the same study, they reported on four other runners besides
Byron. All were free of any evidence of heart disease before
they started running, and all died while running. The lowest
cholesterol level was 228 mg/dl, and all had coronary arteries
severely narrowed or closed with cholesterol deposits. Waller
and Roberts evaluated Bassler's much publicized statement
that marathoners were immune to heart disease, and on the
basis of their evidence, they stated that "Bassler's thesis that
marathon running provides 'immunity to atherosclerosis' is
incorrect." Their conclusion was: "Thus, coronary heart disease appears to be the major killer of conditioned runners aged
40 years and over who die while running."

New Zealander Dennis Stephenson had reason to wish Bas-

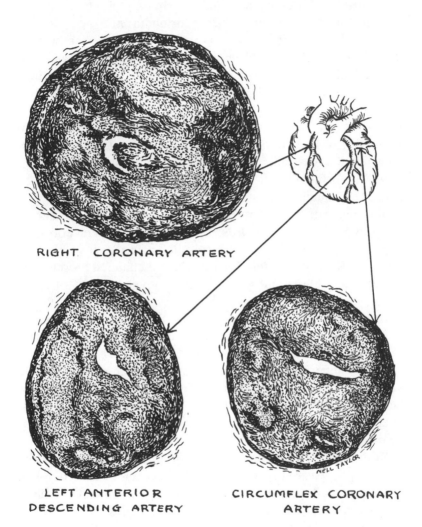

RIGHT CORONARY ARTERY

LEFT ANTERIOR
DESCENDING ARTERY

CIRCUMFLEX CORONARY
ARTERY

CROSS SECTIONS OF CONGRESSMAN BYRON'S
ARTERIES SHOWING EXTENSIVE CLOSURE

(Drawn from photographs provided by William C. Roberts, M. D.,
Natl. Insts. of Health)

sler were right. Despite a lifetime of running in which he held records for 100-mile runs and 24-hour endurance races, he still suffered from heart disease. He died the day after his last marathon. In his early fifties he was very fit, but toward the end he had the same warning signs as Byron: pains in the chest and arm (usually the left arm) and feelings of fatigue in his last marathon.

His autopsy revealed the same coronary cholesterol closures Byron had. If only he had followed a low-cholesterol diet, like his Australian neighbor Rolet de Castella.

It is unfortunate that runners who develop heart disease by eating too much cholesterol and fat are not aware that the symptoms can be reversed. Ron Clarke, former holder of many world running records, at age 45 underwent coronary bypass surgery for his cholesterol-filled arteries. If Clarke had followed Rolet de Castella's example and changed his diet, the chances are 80 percent that he would never have had bypass surgery.

In 1976–77, 64 people came to the Pritikin Centers instead of having bypass surgery, and have now been followed for five years. More than 80 percent never had to have their bypass surgery; 80 percent had angina when they came, but after five years only 30 percent had angina; our deaths in five years for heart disease average only 0.6 percent per year, the lowest ever reported in medical journals for any type of treatment for heart patients like these.

You may not be aware too that of all people who undergo coronary bypass surgery, 10 to 20 percent suffer complete blockage of all their bypasses within the first year. On a high-cholesterol diet, bypasses can close ten times as fast as the original arteries did. It is crucial to go on a low-fat, low-cholesterol diet after bypass surgery.

Jim Shettler's sudden death shocked the running community. Jim had trained like a marathoner since the age of 15. Lean at 6 feet 1 inch and 150 pounds, he had a slow pulse and low blood pressure. He was a nonsmoker and had competed for 25 years in 3,000-meter to 10-mile runs. He had run many marathons. On a day in 1976, at age 42, he ran for three hours over hilly terrain in preparation for his next marathon. The following day, in Oakland, California, he died.

The autopsy was very clear: A main left artery was almost entirely closed with cholesterol deposits. There was little question that this blockage had created a fatal arrhythmia (irregular heartbeat) and sudden death.

If there were any truth in Bassler's statements that 1) marathon runners cannot develop heart disease and 2) if you have heart disease, 10,000 miles of training runs will clean the cholesterol from your arteries, Jim would have been alive. Once again, cholesterol cannot be "burned out" by running or any other exercise. Cholesterol cannot be used for calories or fuel. So to advise runners that because they are active they do not have to watch their cholesterol intake closely is deceptive and dangerous, and I urge you to get your cholesterol under control.

Dr. John Vogel reported on a case identical to Jim Shettler's (*Adv. Cardiol.* Vol. 26, Karger, Basel, 1979, pp. 121–124). A 64-year-old male marathon runner woke up one night just one month after his last marathon with a strange sensation in his chest. He went to a hospital's emergency room, where he developed ventricular fibrillation—an irregular heartbeat in which the rate increases up to 300 beats per minute and the heart stops pumping blood. It means death is imminent. Fortunately, he was revived with emergency measures. An angiogram, or X-ray, of his coronary arteries showed cholesterol deposits narrowing a main left artery by 90 percent. He had immediate bypass surgery, and with the improved blood flow, the arrhythmia disappeared.

The surgeons noted that his right coronary artery was 30 percent closed, but felt the condition wasn't advanced enough to bypass. To protect himself, the patient put himself on many supplements, vitamins E and C, lecithin, brewer's yeast, wheat germ, and so on. He carefully followed Bassler's recommendations and drank beer regularly, and especially after marathons.

Two years later, his treadmill test became abnormal. Another angiogram revealed that the right coronary artery, which had taken 64 years to close 30 percent, had in two years closed 100 percent. In that two-year period, he had run a sub-4-hour marathon.

In 1978, two years later, he was running 10 to 15 miles each day, in preparation for a marathon a month away, when again he went into arrhythmia. He got to the hospital too late, and never regained consciousness. The autopsy revealed that an unbypassed left artery had completely closed, producing a fatal heart attack. This man's dietary supplement program may have been related to the rapid artery closure that finally killed him, since it was the only real change in his lifestyle.

Dr. Thomas Pickering of Cornell University has studied arrhythmias (abnormal heart rhythms) and finds that they occur more frequently during exercise; this, he suggests, could be the principal cause of runners' deaths. He said that a person is at increased risk of arrhythmia death if he runs, and at little risk if he doesn't.

Irwin Baker found that to be true: His arrhythmia almost killed him. When he had been on the Pritikin diet for only six weeks, his arrhythmia had disappeared and he could stop his medication and start running. That was six years ago, and he has run many marathons and ultramarathons since then. Arrhythmia and sudden death in runners could be more closely attributed to the wrong diet.

In 1982 Dr. George Sheehan reported a study that sounded the death knell for Bassler's theory of the invincible runner. "DISHEARTENING NEWS" was the headline, and Sheehan wrote, "Men who have taken up running to prevent a heart attack may find it all a waste of time. A five-year study done at Methodist Hospital in Houston reports that a large proportion of men, aged 40 to 60, who were long-distance runners developed evidence of coronary heart disease."

The 41 subjects in the study had been marathon runners for at least two years before the study began. At the beginning of the investigation, 5 men had positive (abnormal) stress tests; by the end of the third year, 13 had developed positive tests; by the five-year mark, 18 recorded positive stress tests. None of the men had chest pains yet, or other heart-related symptoms, at the end of the five-year study.

When those runners who tested abnormal were checked with the normal runners, there was no difference in average:

1. Miles run per year (1,400);
2. Age (48 years);
3. Cholesterol (192 mg/dl);
4. Bruce treadmill time (12 minutes).

A short time later, three of the abnormal group worsened. One died following a heart attack, another was required to undergo coronary bypass surgery, and the third was confirmed to have heart disease.

Heart disease gradually evolved in all of these men, and in time most of them would show an abnormal stress test, followed by heart attack, angina, and death. Running itself cannot prevent these tragedies.

Rarely is there such an opportunity to observe this closely as the arteries of a healthy runner gradually close through the years. Dr. Jeffrey Handler reported the case of a highly trained marathon runner, a 48-year old marine, who after a one-month period of chest pain checked into the Naval Regional Medical Center in San Diego for evaluation. This man had competed in athletic events since childhood and had begun a vigorous running program eight years before. He was running 50–60 miles a week at an eight-minute-per-mile pace, and before a marathon increased to more than 70 miles per week. Not only had he completed seven marathons, but he had also done 10K runs and 52-mile ultramarathons. Usually he finished in the top 10 percent of his age group.

The angiogram revealed a 99 percent closure of one of his main left arteries with cholesterol deposits, the same as in Jim Shettler's case and with Dr. Vogel's patient.

How could this marine, in superfit condition, a nonsmoker whose cholesterol level was only 185 mg/dl despite the fact that he was on the high-fat and high-cholesterol marine diet, develop heart disease? Dr. Handler comments: "This patient remains the best described example of the failure of a vigorous running program to prevent the progression of coronary atherosclerosis.

"Unfortunately, statements regarding the protective value of running have been made in the medical literature and have been widely circulated among runners. These assertions are not only inaccurate, but potentially dangerous. They foster the tempting illusion of invincibility in the runner."

The marine's blood cholesterol of 185 mg/dl did not prevent cholesterol plaque from closing his arteries. He was perhaps unaware that eating dairy products can keep total cholesterol low while still allowing cholesterol deposits in the artery walls to form the cholesterol boils that eventually prevent blood from reaching part of the heart muscle. His 185 cholesterol level increased his risk of dropping dead of heart disease by five to one compared with the risk if his cholesterol level had been 160.

The Masai are an East African nomadic cattle-herding tribe who exemplify this phenomenon. Milk is the staple of their diet, and the average Masai drinks three to five quarts a day. Yet the average cholesterol level is 135 mg/dl and it was formerly believed that the Masai were safe from coronary heart disease in spite of their high-cholesterol, high-fat diet. However, ten years ago, the hearts and aortae of 50 Masai men, most of whom had been killed in accidents, were collected for autopsy (*Am. J. Epid.* 95:26, 1972). Measurement of the aortae showed extensive atherosclerosis, and the coronary arteries showed thickening equal to that of elderly American males. The blood cholesterol of the Masai is indicative neither of the amount of fat in their diet (66 percent of the 3,000 calories they consume—50 percent higher than the American diet); of their cholesterol intake (600 milligrams—the same as Americans); nor of the degree of atherosclerosis. Why? Because the large quantity of milk they drink artificially lowers the amount of cholesterol found in their blood. Studies suggest that a factor in milk lowers blood cholesterol levels (*Am. J. Clin. Nutr.,* 1974, 27:464–69). While there is a positive correlation between the amount of cholesterol in the blood and the incidence of cardiovascular disease, low cholesterol levels influenced by the consumption of dairy products are misleading and cannot guarantee freedom from disease now or in the future.

Sudden death from ventricular fibrillation is probably the main cause of runners' deaths. In 1958 Dr. Claude Beck of the Cleveland Clinic had studied fibrillation and concluded that it could not occur unless one or more areas of the three coronary arteries and their branches were substantially closed. During periods of little activity, the amount of blood required by the heart is so small that even if one artery is 90-percent closed, the heart looks healthy and pink. But when you exercise vigorously, the heart requires more blood, so if you have an artery closed by 90 percent, the part of the heart nourished by the closed artery turns blue.

This uneven, or checkerboard, distribution of oxygenated blood produces uneven electrical currents, and when the difference in blood flow becomes too great—the faster the heart-rate, the more uneven it will be—ventricular fibrillation is almost inevitable, and almost inevitably fatal.

Dr. Meyer Friedman, cardiologist at Mount Zion Hospital in San Francisco, supports this concept. "The greatest danger," he says, "is the immediate occurrence of arrhythmia, a ventricular fibrillation of the heart—and that's instant death. *That can only affect the people who have serious coronary-artery disease* [my emphasis]. But only 50 percent of the people who died instantaneously during exercise were aware of the fact that they had serious coronary disease. In fact, a study at Johns Hopkins found that 28 percent of heart attack victims had seen a physician within two weeks prior to their deaths (Baltimore study). At autopsy, of course, we find their blood vessels are pretty badly occluded" (*The Jogger,* June 1979).

Some have thought that sheer exhaustion and collapse can precipitate the irregular rhythms of ventricular fibrillation. In the 1968 Olympic Games in Mexico City, the high altitude caused hundreds of participants to collapse. The oxygen deprivation created loss of sight, migraine headaches, nausea and vomiting, blue lips, drop in systolic blood pressure to 60 mm mercury, rapid heartbeat, and other symptoms; but none of the athletes died or developed heart problems. If your heart is free of significant coronary-artery closure, exhaustion does not result in injury.

Too many people die when they exercise more vigorously than usual—when they shovel snow; play tennis, golf, or other sports; or run marathons. Sadly, the running death of Jim Shettler, 42, winner of the National AAU Masters 25K run, heads a steady procession of others who ran for their health but died of their diets.

We remember:

- Jim Dooley, 37, who directed the expansion of the Anaheim stadium for the Los Angeles Rams, died running near his home.
- Robert Clarke, 49, physiologist, died during his daily run.
- Col. Giles Hall, 50, USAF Director of Health Professions Recruiting for the Air Force, a daily jogger for 20 years, died while jogging.
- Dr. Robert Summers, 54, longtime Administrator of the Miami Heart Institute, died while jogging.
- Dr. Edward Lauth, 46, who instituted a jogging program for the American Heart Institute, died while running.

- Dr. David Doroff, 49, psychologist, completed an 18-mile training run for the New York Marathon, had a normal reading in a stress test conducted by his cardiologist, and then dropped dead in the doctor's office. Two of his coronary arteries were 90 percent closed, and the third, 60 percent.
- Duane Armstrong, 59, a five-year member of the Seniors Track Club (California), died while jogging.
- Ron Holmes, 37, a member of the Seniors Track Club, died during the Napa Valley Blossom Time Run. His recent physical had been perfect.
- Dr. Stephen W. Royce, Jr., 51, marathon runner and member of the Seniors Track Club, died in his sleep.
- Richard Peek, 58, marathon runner, died after a 12-mile run.
- Russ Hargreaves, 67, a retired recreation department supervisor, died while running.
- Dodge Parker, 29, player coach of the Orange County (California) Stars of the International Volleyball Association, died of a heart attack.
- Bill English, 19, football player, died of a heart attack.
- Chuck Hughes, 28, Detroit Lions receiver, died of a heart attack.
- Jim Fixx, 52, died while running.
- Jacques Bussereau, 48, died running in the 1984 New York Marathon.

In 1971, before exercise deaths became a subject of national interest, Dr. Ernst Jokl published a monograph on more than 100 cases of sudden death during exercise. Dr. Jokl writes: "The group studied by us is distinguished by the fact that the cardiac diseases had proceeded without symptoms and without impairment of physical fitness. Several of the victims had been outstanding athletes. Among the postmortem findings, coronary atherosclerosis and degenerative changes of the myocardium (heart muscle) were the most frequent. . . .

"Even the most strenuous exercise will not cause death in subjects with normal hearts."

Like to run? Then change your diet! Dr. Paul Thompson reported data from Rhode Island from 1975 to 1980. For each sedentary man 30 to 64 years of age who experienced sudden death, there were seven joggers. Seven jogging sudden deaths to one sedentary sudden death! Dr. Thompson writes: "Exercise contributes to sudden death," and I add: only on the American diet.

If you like to run, great! Your body will benefit immeasurably from the exercise. But please, get your diet under control too. By now you know that the Pritikin Program of proper diet and exercise can pave the way to a long, healthy, vital life. What becomes abundantly clear, however, is that diet and exercise are integral parts of the program, and neither should be undertaken to the exclusion of the other. Now here's how you begin.

———————PART TWO———————

THE RUNNER'S DIET: SEVEN SURVIVAL STAPLES

7

"I Don't Have Time to Cook" Cookery

If you're convinced of the advantages of combining running or any other athletic program with the Pritikin diet, but feel it is not feasible for you because you have so little time for shopping and cooking, this chapter is for you. In these pages you'll find a recommended plan that will enable you to eat Pritikin-style meals day-in, day-out, from the time you take your first bite in the morning until you have your last nibble before retiring at night—and still have enough time for all your other commitments.

The plan can be used to provide you with a scheme for all your meals, should you desire. Of course, you don't have to follow this plan at all in order to adhere to the Pritikin diet and meet your nutritional needs, but doing so can provide you with an easy approach that will minimize your time in the kitchen. To follow the plan, you will need to prepare a few simple staple foods for storage in your refrigerator or freezer. Once they are on hand, you can use them "as is" when you don't feel like cooking. You may also use them as key ingredients, giving you a big head start in preparing a wide variety of interesting recipes when you do have more time to prepare a meal.

Our diet recommendations are based on our years of experience with Pritikin diet cookery of tasty, versatile dishes, and our knowledge of your nutritional needs as a runner or other kind of athlete. At the heart of the plan you will find a pared-down list of seven easily prepared basic foods to keep on hand. The list was developed on the assumption that most readers like to eat some dairy and animal foods as allowed on the Pritikin diet. * If you eat neither (that is, are a very strict vegetarian called a "vegan"), the only nutritional modification you'll need to make is to take some vitamin B_{12} in tablet or other form once every several months.

THE S.S.S. FOOD PLAN

The Seven Survival Staples seem, at first glance, to be a rather odd assortment, but each has earned its exalted place for very good reasons, as you'll soon see. They are: cooked brown rice, cooked dried beans, simmered chicken with stock, tomato veggie stew, mock sour cream, berry-apple compote, and frozen bananas. Cooked brown rice and cooked dried beans have earned top billing for their nutritional value and because hundreds of millions of people in the southern hemisphere and the Orient who subsist on one or both of these foods have evolved unique and tantalizing cuisines utilizing them. We have been able to make convenient and surprisingly good adaptations of some of their dishes.

Cooked from scratch, both brown rice and dried beans take a bit of time—about 45 minutes for the rice and well over an

---

* The Pritikin dietary recommendations are listed in the "Guidelines for following the Pritikin Diet" (page 89) and in the "Foods to Use and to Avoid" chart (pages 97–102).

hour for most beans. But since both keep well and are especially useful in preparing many different dishes, it makes good sense to include them as survival staples in the form of already-cooked foods. Fix a large batch of each once a week, and you're miles ahead in meal preparation.

Simply prepared cooked chicken, made by simmering it in lots of broth, is next on the list. If you aren't a vegetarian, and want to include some animal food in your diet, cooked chicken, sliced or chopped and refrigerated, can be extremely useful. The broth left after cooking the chicken should be defatted and refrigerator- or freezer-stored for later use. We use the liquid in several recipes in the book because it enhances flavor so much. The chicken itself can be used "as is" for sandwiches, or for classic chicken dishes like chicken salad, chicken curry, chicken à la king, chicken tacos, and Chinese stir-fry vegetables with chicken, among others, following our recipe adaptations.

Next on the S.S.S. list is a tomato-based stew made with an assortment of vegetables. The stew can be refrigerated or frozen. You can use it right from the refrigerator as a vegetable relish or even made into a simple green-salad dressing, or serve it hot as a vegetable or a topping over starchy foods such as cooked brown rice, plain baked potato, beans, or whole-wheat pasta. If you wish, you can convert the stew into an authentic-tasting Italian spaghetti sauce with a few simple additions. Or by combining the stew with just one other survival staple, either cooked chicken or cooked dried beans, you can bake delicious casserole dishes, *Chicken Ratatouille* * or *Bean Casserole,* following the simple directions for these recipes.

Store-purchased (or homemade) yogurt containing 1% or less fat, by weight, or a recipe called *Mock Sour Cream,* is another recommended staple. Yogurt and *Mock Sour Cream* are frequently interchangeable, so if you like the taste of yo-

---

* All recipe titles are italicized.

gurt and have an acceptably low-in-fat variety available to you, you can use it in place of *Mock Sour Cream* in most instances. We like *Mock Sour Cream* because it is so versatile in the diet and is easy to make. It keeps well in the refrigerator for days, or can be frozen, then reconstituted by vigorous whipping with a fork. It's excellent as a base for a green-salad dressing, vegetable dip, or sandwich spread, recipes for all of which are provided. It is especially good as a topping for a baked potato, served with chopped chives or scallions.

How do you satisfy a sweet tooth when following the Pritikin diet, without cheating or spending more time than you want preparing a fancy dessert? That's where the frozen bananas and *Berry-Apple Compote* come in! Using frozen bananas, you can make goodies like *Smoothies* or *"Ice Cream"* in a flash. They taste so good, you'll swear they can't be legal! *Berry-Apple Compote* is a simple but inspired recipe. As a topping, it makes a special treat of a fresh fruit cup or combination fresh and frozen fruit cup. Whip a little into some *Mock Sour Cream* (or yogurt) or, for a prettier effect, make the components into a parfait by layering them and ending with a garnish of crushed dry cereal. Or, using beaten egg whites, make a baked fruit meringue with the *Berry-Apple Compote*. Keep some of the compote in your freezer beside a plastic bag filled with ripe, peeled bananas, and you'll never give Häagen-Dazs another thought.

Cooked brown rice, cooked dried beans, simmered chicken, a tomato-based stew with vegetables, *Mock Sour Cream*, frozen bananas, and *Berry-Apple Compote*—there you have them, your Seven Survival Staples—your key to easy, diversified delicious Pritikin meals and even sweet snacks, to accompany your running program.

USING THE SEVEN SURVIVAL STAPLES

The seven staples are at the core of your food plan. Used just as is, and supplemented with green salads and a few fresh fruits, they can fulfill all of your nutritional requirements. You can even use one of them for breakfast as I frequently do. Many mornings I have a bowl of cold cooked brown rice, topped with sliced bananas or other fresh fruit. You can add a little nonfat milk, if you like it moistened.

However, we do suggest you include a few additional foods in your menu plan for variety. Ordinary foods like baked white and sweet potatoes, fresh or frozen corn-on-the-cob, or just lots of good whole-grain bread can round out evening meals, in particular, and make even simple ones very satisfying.

The beauty of the S.S.S. food plan is that it gives you the basics for a highly palatable diet that is optimal for your nutritional needs as a runner. You can use the plan in whatever way suits your day-to-day requirements and individual lifestyle. In its simplest form, you can eat just the staples, or you can use them as starting points in preparing more elaborate meals. The complete list of recipes using the staples as key ingredients (pages 104–108) shows just how interesting your meals can be with this approach.

Naturally, if you wish, you can substitute other appropriate foods for the staples. There may be times when you want a vacation from brown rice, dried beans, simmered chicken, or the other staples, regardless of the many guises in which you've been using them. At these times, you may want to select recipes using other foods from the supplementary recipe section, or you may want to refer to other books on the Pritikin diet, such as *The Pritikin Promise: 28 Days to a Longer, Healthier Life* (Simon & Schuster, 1983), which contains menu suggestions for 28 days complete with a very extensive selection of recipes.

In this book, the recipes include a group of entrées to help you diversify your diet. You'll find, for example, two delicious fish recipes—one for an oven-baked breaded fish, the other for a Creole-style preparation; an easy-to-make pizza (using pita bread); and even a Pritikin-style hamburger. To many of us hamburgers were the sequel to mother's milk in our growing-up years. To be cut off from this culinary invention cold turkey might be asking too much! While our burger doesn't taste just like the fast food version, it's a good-tasting stand-in for the conventional kind when served in a whole-wheat bun, complete with the "fixings"—lettuce, sliced tomato, and onions, and doused with mustard or our *Burger Sauce*.

There's also the possibility that you may want to stay with some of the Seven Survival Staples but not with all of them. Perhaps you like the idea of having cooked rice and simmered chicken on hand but have never liked beans. Or, perhaps you like rice and beans but don't want to bother with the chicken. Whatever the particulars of your situation, you can still use the basic approach behind the S.S.S. food plan—having prepared staples on hand to expedite meal preparation. You may decide to keep on hand five or six of the survival staples recommended, or to add one or two of your own choosing. We think the seven staples together make a uniquely functional group in meal preparation and highly recommend it to you, but the fundamental concept may work better for you in a modified form.

Just remember in planning your meals that most of your calories should come from grains and grain products. Put the emphasis on foods like rice or other grains, bread, cereals, and pasta. The higher-calorie vegetables like potatoes and corn are good, too. Familiarize yourself with the dietary guidelines on page 89 so you have a feeling for the general composition of the diet and the limits on concentrated protein foods in the form of dairy products, beans, chicken or other poultry, fish, or meat.

GUIDELINES FOR FOLLOWING THE PRITIKIN DIET

The diet obtains approximately 80 percent of its total calories from complex carbohydrates,* 10–15 percent from protein, and about 5–10 percent from fat. Cholesterol intake is kept under 100 mg per day. The table compares approximate intake on this diet with intake on the conventional diet.

| | PERCENT OF TOTAL CALORIES | | | CHOLESTEROL |
	FAT	CARB	PROTEIN	(mg/day)
Pritikin Diet	5–10	80	10–15	10–100
Conventional Diet	40–45	45	10–20	600–800

Adhere carefully to the do's and don't's of the table of Foods to Use and to Avoid (pages 97–102) and to the following rules:

1. Eat two or more kinds of whole grain daily (wheat, oats, brown rice, barley, buckwheat, etc.) in the form of cereals, side dishes, pasta, bread, etc.
2. Eat two or more servings of raw vegetable salad and two or more servings of raw or cooked green or yellow vegetables daily, unless you have a tendency to lose weight (see page 114).
3. Eat one piece of citrus fruit and up to three or four fresh fruit servings daily.
4. Eat beans or peas if you wish when meat, fish, or poultry is not eaten. Potatoes may be eaten every day.
5. Limit protein intake from animal sources† as follows: Up to 24 ounces per week of low-fat, low-cholesterol meat, fish, shellfish, or fowl.

* Complex carbohydrates are present in foods as grown, such as whole grains, fresh fruits, and vegetables. On the conventional diet, too few complex carbohydrates are eaten, and much of the carbohydrate consumed is in the form of simple carbohydrates (sugars) or refined carbohydrates, stripped of vitamins, minerals, and fiber.

† Vegetarians eating no animal protein at all may require a supplement of Vitamin B_{12} once every several weeks.

Up to 8 ounces (1 glass) skim milk and 2 ounces of uncreamed cottage cheese per day or equivalent in skim milk products.

6. Egg yolks are to be completely avoided.
7. If you have constipation problems, add some unprocessed wheat bran flakes (starting with 1 tablespoon daily) to your cereal, soup, or other foods.
8. Eat three full meals daily. Don't go hungry between meals; snacks are encouraged. For snacks, eat fruit (not exceeding daily fruit allotment), vegetables and raw salad, or whole-grain bread or crackers that are free of oil, fat, added wheat germ or sweeteners.
9. Flavor with herbs and spices, instead of salt. Keep salt intake minimal.
10. If you need to lose weight, increase vegetables and decrease grains. If you need to gain weight, decrease vegetables and increase grains.

Some Physical Changes You May Notice While Following the Pritikin Diet Suggestions

Within one week, you should notice a change in your bowel habits due to the increased fiber in your diet and to a change in the intestinal bacteria. This may temporarily cause flatulence (gas) and occasional feelings of fullness. Significant health improvements should be noted in one to three months with a lowering of serum cholesterol and blood fats.

Managing Your Weight on the Pritikin Diet

Even though you will be eating mostly carbohydrates (starches) on the Pritikin diet, you can achieve and maintain your ideal weight because you will be consuming much less fat. Foods high in fat are very high in calories; by weight, starches have less than half the calories.

If you wish to lose weight, you can speed up your weight loss by emphasizing the lower calorie foods among those permitted, such as vegetables, and de-emphasizing the higher calorie foods such as grains. If you wish to gain weight, do the reverse. Thus, you would be following the same type of diet whether trying to lose, gain, or maintain weight, except that you would place more or less emphasis on particular foods.

Regardless of whether you are on the regular Pritikin diet or temporarily on a weight loss (700 to 1200 calorie) diet, if you follow the dietary guidelines, you will meet the RDA* for protein † and all other nutrients. Remember that the guidelines are for a new, permanent dietary life-style that will help you to avoid weight problems or problems with degenerative diseases in the future.

Diet During Pregnancy and Lactation

To ensure adequate calcium intake during pregnancy and lactation, a cup or more of broccoli, bok choy, collards, mustard or turnip greens, and/or 2 servings of dairy foods should be eaten daily. If meat, fish, or poultry are omitted, you could increase your intake of dairy foods to 3 to 4 servings without exceeding your protein allotment. Don't habitually use cottage cheese, as it is lower in calcium than other dairy products.

BREAKFASTS

If starting your day with a bowl of cold rice *à la* Nathan Pritikin doesn't send you, how about some cooked cereal? Eaten hot or cold, a cooked cereal has the best staying power,

---

* Recommended Dietary Allowances, established by the National Research Council.

† Because of the reduction in total calorie intake, the percentage of calories from protein will be greater than the usual 12 to 14%.

so that you won't need refueling at 10:00 a.m. We have provided recipes for cooked oatmeal and cooked cracked wheat, and you can also find many suitable whole-grain cereals for cooking available at the supermarket. Preparing hot cereal in the morning doesn't really take that much time. Why not give it a try?

Cold dry cereals don't have quite the staying power of a cooked cereal. If, however, they are your preferred breakfast, make sure you select a brand that gives you the most wholesome product. If you have the time, you can also consider making our *Granola* recipe to use as a dry breakfast cereal or snack food, or eat rolled oats raw (yes, they're very good that way!), gussied up as in our *Apple-Oat Crunch* recipe.

For the additional calories needed by most runners, supplement your breakfast with whole-grain English muffins or bread, toasted, if you desire. Spread them with *Berry-Apple Compote* for a treat, or use a bit of the compote on top of a cooked cereal as a switch from fresh fruit. Nonfat milk and a hot noncaffeine beverage can round out your everyday breakfasts.

For special occasions, or weekends, you might prefer pancakes or "eggs" (egg whites only), made into scrambled or "fried" eggs, using one of the recipes for these dishes.

LUNCHES

If you plan to take lunch with you, sandwiches may be your best bet. On days when you'll be having a vegetarian dinner, you could use the cooked chicken, thinly sliced, on whole-grain bread with lettuce and other raw vegetables, as you like. Sprouts, sliced cucumbers, thinly sliced red onions, and tomatoes all go well with chicken or other kinds of sandwiches, such as those made by converting cooked dried beans, using our recipe, to a simple bean spread. Any of the burgers make good lunchbox items, in a sandwich. Mustard, or our *Mustard-Yogurt Topping,* can be used as sandwich spreads, along with the *Burger Sauce*. Other good choices for packed lunches are cold sweet potatoes, cold corn-on-the-cob, and rice salad made with your number one survival staple—cooked brown rice—or *tabbouli,* another grain-based salad. Recipes for these grain salads are provided. Round out your packed lunch with some raw veggies, one or two pieces of fresh fruit, and a small bag of air-popped popcorn.

On days when you're having lunch at home, the same kinds of foods are just as practical, and, in addition, you have a little more latitude. Why not follow one of the easy recipes for a tasty tostada, made with some of your cooked beans or a leftover bean dish, a *"Fried Egg" Sandwich,* or a Mexican recipe with beans and eggs—*Huevos Rancheros*. Are there leftover baked white or sweet potatoes in the refrigerator? Make delicious mock *"French Fries"* and sweet potato tidbits by peeling and slicing them, then placing the slices on a non-stick cookie sheet to bake in a hot oven until brown. If you're really in a hurry, you can make the simplest sandwich in Pritikin cookery—cut a banana in lengthwise slices and eat it between two pieces of whole-grain bread!

DINNERS

For most people, a satisfying dinner is very important. To assist you with some ideas for dinners, we've provided a few sample menus, some based on the survival staples, and others not. The menus include both quick meals and more elaborate ones. You'll find them on pages 125–128.

Remember, in planning dinners, the more complex-carbohydrate foods the better. It's time to break away from the idea that we should have only one starchy food at a meal. Even if you're already planning on having a rice dish or pasta, feel free to add simply prepared foods like baked potatoes and baked yams or sweet potatoes to any menu. These delicious tubers taste surprisingly good when eaten right along with many rice, bean, or pasta dishes. Many runners on the Pritikin diet bake white potatoes and sweet potatoes or yams for dinner routinely. Put them into the oven together, since they require approximately the same baking time and temperature. If they don't get eaten, they're real assets when stored in the refrigerator for tomorrow's lunch or dinner.

By emphasizing complex-carbohydrate foods like potatoes, grain, bread, corn, and pasta, you'll be giving yourself the best possible nutrition for your needs as a runner, and along the way, you will minimize your intake of foods that are high in fat and cholesterol. You'll also keep your protein intake where it belongs—not too high, not too low.

SNACKS

Eating whenever you're hungry is good Pritikin-diet protocol. The idea is to provide a continuous stream of energy from complex-carbohydrate sources. A few slices of whole-grain bread or some whole-grain crackers is the simplest way to feed a between-meal hunger pang. Just make sure that you select foods that are "legal" by Pritikin guidelines. The table of Foods to Use and to Avoid, pages 97 to 102, gives you the information you need to help make proper selections. Air-popped popcorn, oven-toasted corn tortillas, and fresh fruit are other good, simple snacks. A nutlike snack food can be made with cooked, then baked garbanzo beans, using our recipe. Dips and spreads made with *Mock Sour Cream* or cooked beans, both survival staples, also make wonderful snack foods. If it's something sweet you're craving, look to two other survival staples, frozen bananas and the *Berry-Apple Compote,* for the many delights they can provide, including those terrific *Smoothies!*

BEVERAGES

Coffee, Tea, Chocolate, and Cola Drinks

These beverages contain caffeine or caffeinelike substances called methylxanthines. This can be a particular problem for women, as a number of researchers believe they are related to fibrocystic breast disease. Dr. John P. Minton of Ohio State University treats women with fibrocystic breast disease by eliminating coffee, tea, chocolate, and cola drinks from their diets. Most of his patients recover in a few months. The breasts lose their tenderness, swelling, and discomfort, and the cysts gradually disappear.

The day after you eliminate caffeine from your diet, you may have a minor headache and a feeling of uneasiness. If you were a heavy consumer, your headaches may intensify on the third and fourth days, but on the fifth and sixth days they will gradually disappear. Most people can tolerate the discomfort, but if it gets too much, take headache tablets, especially before bed, so you can get a good night's sleep.

As soon as these transient symptoms are gone, you'll feel a new calmness. Your heart will beat more slowly, and you'll be less uptight about things. If you're accustomed to the pick-me-up of coffee, for a few days you may feel tired in the morning, but by the end of a week you should be free of addiction to caffeine.

To replace caffeine-based hot drinks at the Pritikin Longevity Centers, we serve Postum and two herb teas, Chamomile and Red Bush. Salt-free seltzer, alone or mixed with a little fruit juice, makes a refreshing cold drink. Some people have discovered that just plain water, hot or cold, satisfies that desire for a drink with meals or at other times.

Alcohol

Alcohol is a sensitive subject. If you can abstain, fine! If you must have some, then limit yourself to one beer or glass of wine four times a week. Mixed cocktails have, in general, about half again as much alcohol, so if they are your preferred drink, two or three times a week should be your limit.

The following table will help you choose foods in allowed quantities to supplement your new diet plan and avoid those that are not good for you.

Next let's move on to see exactly how you can get started on the Pritikin diet for runners and athletes.

FOODS TO USE AND TO AVOID ON THE MAINTENANCE DIET

CATEGORY	FOODS PERMITTED	QUANTITY PERMITTED	FOODS TO AVOID
FATS, OILS	None.		All fats and oils, including butter, margarine, shortening, lard, meat fat, all oils, lecithin (as in vegetable spray).
EGGS	Egg whites.	7 per week max. (Raw: two per week max.)	Egg yolks. Fish eggs: caviar, shad roe, etc.
POULTRY, FISH, SHELLFISH* AND MEAT	Chicken, turkey, Cornish game hen (white meat preferred; remove skin). Lean round or flank steak, all visible fat removed. Lean fish, squid and shellfish.	Limit acceptable poultry, fish, and meat to 3½ oz. per day, maximum 1½ lbs. per week. Lobster, oysters, clams, scallops, squid, and mussels: 3½ oz. per day. Shrimp and crab: 1¼ oz. per day. (Replaces entire daily allotment of poultry, fish, or meat.)	Fatty poultry: duck, goose, etc. Fatty fish such as mackerel, sardines, and fish canned in oil. Fatty meats: marbled steaks, fatty hamburger and other fatty ground meat, bacon, spareribs, sausage, frankfurters, luncheon meat, etc. Organ meats: liver, kidneys, hearts, sweetbreads. Smoked, charbroiled, or barbecued foods.

* Our revised recommendations are based on a conservative interpretation of the newest data concerning cholesterol and other possibly atherogenic sterols in shellfish.

FOODS TO USE AND TO AVOID ON THE MAINTENANCE DIET (*cont.*)

CATEGORY	FOODS PERMITTED	QUANTITY PERMITTED	FOODS TO AVOID
DAIRY FOODS	Nonfat (skim) milk, nonfat buttermilk (1% fat, or less, by weight). (8 oz. = one serving)	2 servings/day.	Cream, half-and-half, whole milk and lowfat milk or products containing or made from them, such as sour cream, lowfat yogurt, etc.
	Nonfat yogurt (1% fat, or less, by weight). (8 oz. = one serving)		Nondairy substitutes: creamers, whipped toppings, etc.
	Nonfat (skim) powdered milk. (5 tablespoons = 1 serving)		Cheeses containing over 1% fat by weight.
	Evaporated skim milk. (4 oz. = 1 serving)		
	100% skim milk cheese, primarily uncreamed cottage cheese such as hoop cheese or dry curd cottage cheese or cheeses up to 1% fat by weight. (2 oz. = 1 serving)		
	Sap Sago (Green) cheese.	1–2 oz. per week max.	

GRAINS	All whole or lightly milled grains; rice, barley, buckwheat, millet, etc. Breads, cereals, crackers, pasta, tortillas, baked goods and other grain products without added fats, oils, sugars, or egg yolks.	Not limited. Limit refined grains and grain products (i.e., with bran and germ removed) such as white flour, white rice, white pasta, etc.	Added wheat germ. Grain products made with added fats, oils, sugars, or egg yolks. Bleached white flour; soy flour.
BEANS, PEAS	All beans and peas, tofu.	4 oz. tofu, ½ cup cooked soy beans or 1½ cups other cooked beans or peas can be substituted either for your daily allotment of DAIRY FOODS or POULTRY, FISH, SHELLFISH AND MEAT. Avoid on other days except for small amounts in soups, salads, or other dishes.*	Canned beans with fat.
VEGETABLES	All vegetables except avocadoes and olives.	Limit vegetables high in oxalic acid such as spinach, beet leaves, rhubarb, and swiss chard.	Avocadoes, olives.

* If less than 1,500 calories are consumed, dairy products should not be omitted unless one cup of collard, mustard, turnip, or other dark greens are eaten.

99

FOODS TO USE AND TO AVOID ON THE MAINTENANCE DIET (cont.)

CATEGORY	FOODS PERMITTED	QUANTITY PERMITTED	FOODS TO AVOID
FRUITS,* FRUIT JUICE, SWEETENERS	All fresh fruits.	5 servings per day max.	Cooked, canned, or frozen fruit with added sugars. Products containing added sugars such as: jams, jellies, fruit spreads, and syrups. Fruit juices with added sugar.
	Unsweetened cooked, canned, puréed, or frozen fruit.	1½ lb. per week max.	
	Dried fruit.	1 oz. per day max.	
	Unsweetened fruit juices.	½ cup per day max. *or*	
	Frozen concentrates, undiluted.	2 tbsp. per day max. *or*	
	Barley malt.	1 tbsp. per day max.	Extracted sugars.
DESSERTS OR SNACKS	Dessert and snack items without fats, oils, sugars, or egg yolks.	Plain gelatin (unflavored); one oz. per week max.	Desserts and snack items containing fats, oils, sugars, or egg yolks such as: most bakery goods, packaged gelatin desserts and puddings, candy, chocolate and gum.

* If triglycerides are above 125 mg %, eat only fresh fruit in permitted amount.

NUTS, SEEDS	Chestnuts.	Not limited.	All nuts (except chestnuts). All seeds (except in small quantities for seasoning as with spices).
SALT*	Salt.	Limit salt intake to 4 grams (1,600 mg. sodium) or less per day. Eliminate table salt and restrict the use of high salt or sodium (Na) foods such as soy sauce, pickles, most condiments, prepared sauces, dressings, canned vegetables, and MSG (monosodium glutamate).	Salt from all sources in excess of permitted amount.
CONDIMENTS, SALAD DRESSINGS, SAUCES, GRAVIES, AND SPREADS	Wines for cooking. Natural flavoring extracts. Products without fats, oils, sugars, or egg yolks.	Dry wine preferable. Moderate use.	Products containing fats, oils, sugars, or egg yolks such as: mayonnaise, prepared sandwich spreads, prepared gravies and sauces and most seasoning mixes, salad dressings, catsups, pickle relish, chutney, etc.

* Normal salt (sodium) needs are provided by foods in their natural state. Additional intake should be kept to a minimum.

FOODS TO USE AND TO AVOID ON THE MAINTENANCE DIET (cont.)

CATEGORY	FOODS PERMITTED	QUANTITY PERMITTED	FOODS TO AVOID
BEVERAGES	Mineral water, carbonated water.	Limit varieties with added sodium.	Alcoholic beverages.
	Nonfat (skim) milk or nonfat buttermilk.	See restrictions under DAIRY FOODS above.	Milk containing more than 1% fat by weight.
	Unsweetened fruit juices.	See restrictions under FRUIT above.	Beverages with added sugar or artificial sweeteners.
	Vegetable juices.	Unlimited.	Highly salted juices.
	Herb teas: Red Bush, Chamomile tea preferred. Coffee substitutes: Postum preferred.	2 cups per day.	Beverages with caffeine: coffee, black tea, cola drinks, etc. Decaffeinated coffee.

8

Putting the S.S.S. Food Plan Into Practice

Getting started in a new way of cooking and eating is a little like getting going on a long run. At the start, it seems quite impossible that your heart, lungs, and muscles will sustain you for so many miles, and that it will, in fact, become easier after about the first ten minutes. In like fashion, once you've warmed up to incorporating the S.S.S. food plan into your life, it gets easier and easier, and more rewarding, too.

Step I: Menu Planning

Study the chart of the Seven Survival Staples and the recipes that can be made from them on pages 104–108 to get you started thinking about foods you can prepare after you've started on the S.S.S. food plan. Your own needs and experiences with the recipes will eventually be your best guide to formulating menu plans, but for now you may also get some ideas from the dinner menu plans on pages 125–128.

Use this chart as a guide to make maximum use of the Seven Survival Staples. The page numbers for preparing the staples are shown beside the name of each staple in the left-hand column; recipes that use the prepared staples as important ingredients are listed with their page numbers in the middle column; and additional uses for the prepared staples are suggested in the right-hand column.

STAPLE/PAGE	RECIPES USING PREPARED STAPLES/ PAGE	ADDITIONAL USES
COOKED BROWN RICE/116	*Chinese "Fried" Rice/132* *Spanish Rice/133* *Mexican Rice/133* *Hawaiian Rice/134* *Indian Rice/135* *Rice-Bulgur Pilaf/136* *Confetti Rice/135* *Tuna-Rice Bake/137* *Salmon-Rice Patties/138* *Lentil Patties/148* *Chicken Tacos* or *Enchiladas/151* and *152* *Rice Salad/182* *Fruited Rice Salad/182* *Tropical Tuna Salad/184* *Three-Grain Pancakes/202* *Rice Pudding/213*	1. Accompaniment for other foods; 2. base for beans, sauces, and other foods; 3. cold breakfast cereal or snack, mixed with fresh diced fruit and sprinkled with cinnamon, and served with nonfat milk, if desired.

STAPLE/PAGE	RECIPES USING PREPARED STAPLES/ PAGE	ADDITIONAL USES
COOKED DRIED BEANS/117	*Barrego Beans/139* *Bean Enchiladas/140* *Bean Casseroles/139* *Tacos, Tostadas, and Burritos/142* *Pasta e Fagioli/144* *Bean/Bulgur Combo/145* *Chili/146* *Minestrone/177* *Chef's Salad with Tuna and Beans/178* *Huevos Rancheros/143* *Bean Spread/196* *Hummus Dip/197* *Garbanzo Nuts/216*	1. Toss some in mixed green salads.
SIMMERED CHICKEN AND CHICKEN STOCK/118	*Chinese "Fried" Rice/132* *Chicken Curry/149* *Chicken à la King/150* *Chicken Ratatouille/148* *Chicken Tacos/151* *Chicken Enchiladas/152* *Chinese Stir-Fry Vegetables with Chicken/153* *Chicken Crêpes with White Sauce/154* *Chicken and Okra Gumbo/ 156* *Chicken Salad/185*	1. Slice chicken for chicken sandwiches; 2. use chicken stock as liquid ingredient to enhance flavor in many recipes in book (e.g., *Chicken Curry, Mushroom Cream Sauce,* and others).

STAPLE/PAGE	RECIPES USING PREPARED STAPLES/ PAGE	ADDITIONAL USES
TOMATO/VEGGIE STEW/120	*Bean Casseroles/139* *Chicken Ratatouille/148* *Spaghetti Sauce with Tomato-Veggie Stew/ 164* *Tuna-Rice Bake/137*	1. Topping for rice, beans, baked potatoes, or pasta; 2. hot vegetable; 3. topping for vegetables, such as cabbage, corn kernels, green beans, or greens; 4. enchilada sauce (add chile powder); 5. cold, as vegetable relish or as salad dressing (process in blender and add vinegar).
MOCK SOUR CREAM/121	*Stuffed Baked Potatoes/ 191* *Cucumbers with Mock Sour Cream/179* *Cole Slaw/180* *Creamy Artichoke Dressing/192* *Thousand Island Dressing/ 193* *Onion Dip or Spread/195* *Devilled Egg Dip or Spread/196*	1. Topping for baked potatoes (plain, or mixed with onion powder and served with chopped scallions or chives); 2. topping for green salad (plain, or mixed with lemon juice or herb-flavored vinegar);

STAPLE/PAGE	RECIPES USING PREPARED STAPLES/ PAGE	ADDITIONAL USES
MOCK SOUR CREAM *(cont.)*		3. topping for fresh or fresh- and frozen-fruit cup (plain, or sweetened with fruit juice or blended with fresh fruit).
BERRY-APPLE COMPOTE/122	*Berry-Apple Compote Meringue/208* *Berry-Apple Compote "Ice Cream"/213*	1. Dessert, or topping for fresh fruit cup or fresh- and frozen-fruit cup —plain, or mixed with *Mock Sour Cream* or yogurt (1% or less fat, by weight). (Can be made into a parfait by alternating layers of compote and yogurt or *Mock Sour Cream* and ending with a garnish of crushed dry cereal.) 2. Topping for breakfast toast; 3. gelatinized for a party mold (use plain unflavored gelatin);

STAPLE/PAGE	RECIPES USING PREPARED STAPLES/ PAGE	ADDITIONAL USES
BERRY-APPLE COMPOTE *(cont.)*		4. *cranberry-apple compote* may be used as a relish accompanying sliced turkey or chicken.
FROZEN BANANAS/123	*Smoothies/214* "*Ice Cream*"/213	1. Slice, and top with *Mock Sour Cream,* yogurt (1% or less fat, by weight), *Berry-Apple Compote,* or a combination of the compote and yogurt or *Mock Sour Cream.*

Step II: Shopping

Make a list (see the charts on pages 109–111) and shop for foods you'll need for the S.S.S. food plan. When you've laid in a good supply of nonperishables, like rice, beans, canned tomato products, and spices, your future shopping expeditions should be short and sweet.

SEVEN SURVIVAL STAPLES SHOPPING LIST

To prepare the Seven Survival Staples, you'll need to have on hand all the foods listed in the "Items Needed" column, as well as a few miscellaneous items and items of produce listed at the end of the shopping list. If you have enough storage space, it's convenient to buy larger quantities than the amounts shown, especially of items that store well, such as the rice, beans, and canned tomato products.

SURVIVAL STAPLE	ITEMS NEEDED/SUGGESTED QUANTITIES		COMMENTS
Cooked Brown Rice (page 116)	Raw brown rice	two pounds	Buy bulk or packaged rice. Long-grain variety preferred by most people. Don't buy instant or other parboiled types.
Cooked Dried Beans (page 117)	Dry beans	two pounds	Buy bulk or packaged beans. Pinto beans are a good starting choice, but later on you may wish to try others such as red beans or kidney beans.
Simmered Chicken and Chicken Stock (page 118)	For one recipe: one pkg. chicken thighs	about two and one half pounds	Recipe also requires celery, onions, carrots, and bay leaves. (See *Miscellaneous Shopping List*.)
	one pkg. chicken breasts	about two pounds	
	one pkg. chicken wings	about two pounds	
	one pkg. chicken necks or backs	about one pound	

SEVEN SURVIVAL STAPLES SHOPPING LIST (*cont.*)

SURVIVAL STAPLE	ITEMS NEEDED/SUGGESTED QUANTITIES	COMMENTS
Tomato-Veggie Stew (page 120)	For one recipe: one 28-ounce can crushed tomatoes one 28-ounce can tomato purée one 6-ounce can tomato paste	Recipe also requires celery, onions, green pepper, eggplant, zucchini, and garlic, and Italian seasoning and oregano. (See *Miscellaneous Shopping List*.)
Mock Sour Cream (page 121)	16-ounce container of cottage cheese (1% fat or less, by weight) one quart buttermilk (1% fat or less, by weight), preferred	Recipe also requires lemon juice or vinegar. (See *Miscellaneous Shopping List*.)
Berry-Apple Compote (page 122)	12-ounce bag of frozen cherries, strawberries, or cranberries one 16-ounce can frozen apple juice concentrate	Recipe also requires apples, vanilla and lemon extracts, and cornstarch. (See *Miscellaneous Shopping List*.) Each recipe uses one 12-ounce bag of frozen fruit.
Frozen bananas (page 123)	Bananas (one-half dozen or more)	Select bananas not yet fully ripe, and let them finish ripening at home before peeling and freezing them (unless you can find fully-ripened bananas ready to freeze that are free of bruises).

MISCELLANEOUS SHOPPING LIST
FOR ENTIRE GROUP:

PRODUCE/SEASONING AND STAPLES	NEEDED FOR
two pounds onions two carrots one bunch celery	*Simmered Chicken* and *Chicken Stock* or *Tomato-Veggie Stew*
one large green pepper one small eggplant two medium zucchini one bulb garlic	*Tomato-Veggie Stew*
four apples	*Berry-Apple Compote*
one lemon (or vinegar)	*Mock Sour Cream*
vinegar (or fresh lemon)	*Mock Sour Cream*
cornstarch, vanilla extract, and lemon extract	*Berry-Apple Compote*
Italian seasoning, oregano	*Tomato-Veggie Stew*
bay leaves	*Simmered Chicken* and *Chicken Stock*

Step III: Preparing the Seven Survival Staples

Recipes for the Seven Survival Staples and instructions for their preparation follow on pages 116–124. But before preparing any recipes, please read the "Important Points about the Recipes" on pages 128 and 129, pertaining to procedures and ingredients you'll be using.

When and how to get started on the food plan is an individual matter, but for many people the most convenient time to prepare the staples is on the weekend, when they have a little more leisure time. Here's a plan of action that you may like.

Before starting an early run, put the dried beans up to soak, following the recipe instructions. When you return to the kitchen later in the day, put them on the stove to cook. Next rinse and skin the chicken, and after it is cooking on the stove, start the rice in its pot. With all three pots simmering merrily away, begin to prep the vegetables for the *Tomato-Veggie Stew*. Cooking the stew is a snap, but the prepping of the vegetables will take some time if you don't have a food processor to speed up the cutting of the vegetables. When the beans, rice, *Tomato-Veggie Stew,* and chicken breasts, thighs, and stock have finished cooking, let them cool a little, then store in the refrigerator. If you've made enough, you may want to stash part of your yield in plastic zip-lock bags in the freezer, first deboning the chicken to save space, if you wish. The chicken stock should be refrigerated overnight to permit the fat to harden so that it can be skimmed off the top. Then measure the stock into plastic bags or other containers for storage.

If you have time left, complete the preparation of the staples by making the *Berry-Apple Compote* and *Mock Sour Cream,* two easy recipes, and store some peeled bananas in a large zip-lock bag in the freezer. You can also freezer-store the compote or *Mock Sour Cream,* if you wish. Now stand back and congratulate yourself, and, if you're hungry, sample or sup on your creations!

If this all-day cooking orgy seems an entirely impractical approach for you, you could prepare a few of the staples at a time, gradually easing into the S.S.S. food plan. Whatever you decide, remember, it gets easier as you go along. After the initial preparation of all the staples, you can just replenish them one by one, as you run out. In addition, you'll be generating leftovers from interesting recipes made from the staples as time goes on. These, stored in your refrigerator or freezer, provide the basis for many quick meals.

COOKING THE S.S.S. FOOD PLAN FOR OTHERS

If others, besides yourself, will be eating your food, you may be concerned about its appropriateness for growing children, pregnant women, nursing mothers, or elderly people. The Seven Survival Staples, augmented by salads made with dark green lettuce and citrus and other fresh fruits, can provide all of our nutritional requirements at any stage of life. However, the Seven Survival Staples are meant as a minimalist approach to eating. They can be expanded with an infinite variety of foods used on the Pritikin diet, using the Pritikin guidelines as directions, and keeping in mind varying caloric requirements for different individuals as determined by size, age, amount of activity, and other factors.

THE S.S.S. FOOD PLAN AND YOUR WEIGHT

Most runners and other endurance athletes need to eat large quantities of high-calorie complex carbohydrate foods to provide themselves with enough calories. So most readers can stow away large amounts of such foods in the form of bread, cereals, and other grains, beans, and higher-calorie vegetables such as corn, and maintain an optimal weight.

But perhaps you've just started running and have a few pounds to lose. To expedite your weight loss, the only modification you'll need to make is to eat smaller quantities of these higher-calorie complex carbohydrate foods, and to supplement them with lots of bulky, low-calorie complex carbohydrates in the form of green salads, soups, and plain steamed vegetables. If you can, eat a large green salad twice a day, making sure that it includes plenty of dark green lettuce. The darker green varieties are preferred on the Pritikin diet to iceberg or other light green lettuces. Because soups have a watery base, they are, in general, a good way to fill up without getting a large number of calories. The *Italian Peasant Soup* (page 176) would be a good choice for you, but omit the bread used with the soup. You can make the recipe for another soup, *Minestrone* (page 177), less caloric by adding fewer beans, or by thinning with a little extra liquid to reduce the calories per serving. Among the Seven Survival Staples, the recommended food for dieters to be eaten without restriction is the *Tomato-Veggie Stew,* so prepare large amounts of it. Use the stew by itself or on top of plain low-calorie steamed vegetables, such as cabbage wedges, green beans, or greens like kale, bok choy, or mustard, turnip, or collard greens. Or, put *gobs* of *Tomato-Veggie Stew* on *small* amounts of pasta, rice, or other higher-calorie foods.

A more common problem with runners who go on the Pritikin diet is the danger of losing too much weight! This happens when runners who are at their optimal weight emphasize lower-calorie complex carbohydrate foods. They think that when they are on the Pritikin diet they need to eat lots of large green salads, soups, and plain steamed vegetables, and they don't eat enough of the higher-calorie complex carbohydrate foods, like breads and grains. This point cannot be stressed too much:

> *Make sure you are eating plenty of higher-calorie complex carbohydrates, and if your weight begins to drop below the optimal, cut back on salads, soups, and low-calorie vegetables, and increase your intake of high-calorie breads, grains, beans, and high-calorie vegetables.*

9

Recipes

THE SEVEN SURVIVAL STAPLES

After you've assembled the raw materials for making the
Seven Survival Staples, you're ready to prepare them for use
in the S.S.S. food plan. Here's how to go about it, beginning
with your number one survival staple.

COOKED BROWN RICE

While all seven survival staples have a uniquely valuable
purpose in the S.S.S. food plan, cooked brown rice leads in
importance because it carries a large part of the nutritional
and caloric load. Always keep in mind that unrefined grains,
such as brown rice, are recommended for the bulk of your
calories on the Pritikin diet. When on hand already cooked,
brown rice can quickly step into a variety of roles as the base
or accompaniment for other foods, or as an ingredient in many

delicious recipes. The complete list of recipes using cooked brown rice as an ingredient is shown on the chart showing how to use the Seven Survival Staples (page 104).

The long-grain variety of brown rice is usually preferred for its lighter texture and more attractive appearance, but if you like the equally nutritious short-grain variety, you can use the same method to prepare it. Experiment a bit to find just the right pot for cooking your rice. It might even be worthwhile to invest in a new pot just for that purpose. If your refrigerator is roomy enough, you can then store the rice in the refrigerator right in the pot. We like to cook and store our rice in a large stainless-steel skillet with a tight-fitting lid. Since rice keeps at least a week, you may want to double this recipe to have more on hand. It takes no longer to cook and you will more than likely use it up before the week is over.

    3 cups water
    1½ cups washed brown rice

Bring the water to a boil, add rice slowly and return to a boil. Cover and reduce heat to low. Cook for 40–45 minutes, covered, without stirring the rice. The rice should be cooked when there is no more steam escaping from under the lid. Fluff before serving.

Makes about 4½ or 5 cups.

Note: How to Reheat Cooked Brown Rice.

If you are putting a hot sauce or other hot food, such as hot cooked beans, on top of the rice, you may not wish to bother reheating it. But if you are using rice as an accompaniment, most people prefer it hot. Here are two methods for reheating cooked brown rice.

Oven Method: Place desired quantity of rice in a baking dish, cover, and place in a 325° to 375° oven to heat through.

A small quantity of rice—1 to 3 cups—should be sufficiently hot after about 10–15 minutes of heating, but larger amounts may require a little longer.

Steamer Method: Fit a steamer basket into a pot of boiling water. Place rice to be reheated in the basket, cover and let steam for about 10 minutes or until heated through.

COOKED DRIED BEANS

There are many dried beans to choose from, but a good one to get started with is the little speckled pinto bean that turns a lovely red when cooked. The plain cooked beans may be eaten just by themselves, perhaps with a dash of bottled hot sauce, or you may use them in preparing many different kinds of recipes. You'll find an interesting array of recipes using cooked beans on pages 138–147.

To cook any dried bean, follow the general procedure described below, including the presoaking period that shortens cooking time and tenderizes the beans. Many cooks discard the water in which the beans were soaked and replace it with fresh water for cooking. The advantage is a *small* reduction in the substances (oligosaccharides) that cause flatulence, or gas, in some people, but you will also lose some nutrients, flavor, and color. If you wish, you can store beans in the refrigerator right in the cooking pot, or transfer them to other containers. Beans keep in the refrigerator for about a week, or you may freeze them.

3–8 cups dried beans, washed and picked over
2½ cups water per cup of beans

Place the beans in a pot large enough to accommodate them, as they swell to about double their size. Use a fast-soak method as follows: Bring the water to a boil, let the beans cook for 5–10 minutes, turn off the heat, and let the beans soak, covered, for ½ to 1 hour.

To cook, add water to cover the beans by at least an inch. Bring to a boil, turn down heat, and simmer covered (watch to avoid boiling over) or with lid ajar until the beans are tender but not mushy. Cooking time will vary from about 1 hour to 2 hours, depending upon the kind of bean you're cooking. Some approximate cooking times for a few favorites: 1½–2 hours for pinto beans, 1½ hours for red beans, 1 hour for kidney beans, and 2 hours for garbanzo beans.

If you plan to cook beans for tacos, tostadas, burritos, or enchiladas, or just to eat them over brown rice, a highly recommended alternate method is to cook the beans following the procedure described above, adding seasonings to the water when starting the cooking period. The finished beans can then be used in any of the corn tortilla-based dishes in the recipe section, or simply over rice, without additional seasoning. A variety of seasonings may be added to the cooking water, according to your preferences, but one very simple seasoning method is to add lots of garlic cloves and canned green chile salsa. If cooking pinto beans (an ideal bean for these uses), for each pound of beans (about 2½ cups), add 2–3 chopped garlic cloves and one 7-ounce can green chile salsa.

SIMMERED CHICKEN AND CHICKEN STOCK

This recipe yields a bonus. Besides the flavorful chicken it makes, which you can use just as is or in a variety of interesting recipes (pages 148–156), you'll have prepared about two quarts of strong chicken stock that can be used to enhance the flavor of many dishes. Chicken stock, in fact, is the preferred liquid ingredient in many recipes in this book. To prepare this double-purpose recipe, purchase packages of chicken breasts, thighs, necks or backs, and wings, in approximately the amounts shown below. The necks, backs, and wings will intensify the flavor of the stock but are not saved. Instructions for storing the stock and cooked chicken are provided in the recipe directions.

    1 package chicken thighs (approximately 2–2½ pounds)
    1 package chicken breasts (approximately 2 pounds)
    1 package chicken wings (approximately 1¾–2 pounds)
    1 package chicken necks or backs (approximately 1 pound)
    3 stalks celery with tops
    1 onion, unpeeled and quartered
    2 carrots
    2 bay leaves
    3 quarts water

Remove the skin and pockets of fat from the chicken thighs and breasts. Rinse all the chicken parts. Place the thighs and breasts only in a steamer basket or colander that can be fitted into the pot. The thighs and breasts will be covered by the liquid, then removed after they have simmered long enough to make them tender. The wings, necks, and backs will need to cook longer to make the stock stronger.

Put the wings, necks, backs, vegetables, and water in the pot. Insert the steamer basket or colander into the pot, making sure that the thighs and breasts are covered by the water, and bring the water to a boil. Cover the pot, turn down the heat, and let the liquid simmer for about 45 minutes. Remove the steamer basket with the thighs and breasts, and let the chicken cool. Let the stock continue simmering, covered, for another 1¼–1½ hours.

Refrigerate the thighs and breasts after they have cooled a little, and when thoroughly chilled, remove the meat from the bones, if desired. Store the boned or unboned chicken in small plastic zip-lock containers in the refrigerator or freezer. If you wish, the chilled chicken may be sliced for sandwiches or cut into chunks before putting it into the plastic bags. If chicken will not be used in the next few days, it should be frozen.

Pour the chicken stock from the pot through cheesecloth or Handi-Wipes into a suitable container, pressing down or squeezing to get all the stock to drain through. Discard the wings, necks, backs, and vegetables. Let stock refrigerate overnight until the fat has hardened on the top, then remove fat completely and pour stock into small plastic zip-lock bags. Store the stock in the freezer.

Makes approximately one dozen chicken thighs and breasts and about two quarts chicken stock.

TOMATO-VEGGIE STEW

This vegetable stew has earned its place as one of the Seven Survival Staples because it can be used in so many appetizing ways. We've praised its versatility elsewhere, but it's hard to overstate the utility of a dish that can serve as a cold relish; hot vegetable; sauce or topping for pasta, rice, beans, or potatoes; or as a casserole ingredient. Two excellent oven casseroles using *Tomato-Veggie Stew* are *Chicken Ratatouille,* which combines the stew with chunks of simmered chicken— nothing else added—and *Oven Bean Casserole,* in which the stew is simply mixed with cooked dried beans. This adaptable dish can even be quickly converted to a spaghetti sauce (recipe on page 164) or a green-salad dressing, by processing it through a blender and adding a little vinegar to taste. Here it is:

          1 onion, quartered
          3 large cloves garlic
          1 28-ounce can crushed tomatoes
          1 28-ounce can tomato purée
          1 6-ounce can tomato paste
          2 cups celery, diced very fine
       1½ cups onion, diced

1 large green pepper, diced
1 small eggplant, diced small
2 medium zucchini, diced
1 tablespoon Italian herb seasoning
1 teaspoon oregano

Place the quartered onion, garlic, and about a third to a half of the crushed tomatoes and tomato purée in a blender; blend well. Stir in the tomato paste and blend again. Transfer blender ingredients to a pot, and add the rest of the canned tomato products and all the vegetables and seasonings. Bring to a boil, lower heat, and let simmer uncovered for 45 to 50 minutes.

Note: To prepare the stew, cut the vegetables by hand or, if you prefer, use a food processor or blender for the onions, celery, and green pepper. Avoid cutting them too finely. As a variation, you might try cutting the vegetables in larger chunks. The smaller-size chunks, though, give the stew a desirable sauce-like quality. You can also vary the stew by using other vegetables, such as yellow crook-neck or scalloped squash.

If you like, cook the stew in a crock pot or in the oven in an oven casserole. *Tomato-Veggie Stew* keeps well in the refrigerator for about a week, and you may freeze it.

Makes about 2½ quarts.

MOCK SOUR CREAM

Mock Sour Cream, an easily made nonfat dairy concoction, can add lots of interest to your S.S.S. food plan. Use it just like sour cream as a baked potato topping, or vary its consistency to use as the base of wonderful spreads, dips, and dressings. Unlike yogurt, which it resembles in some ways, the consistency of *Mock Sour Cream* is changeable. It tends to thicken after being stored in the refrigerator for several days or after freezing. Just thin it down by whipping in a little nonfat milk, or yogurt or buttermilk that is 1% or less fat, by weight, straining the buttermilk to remove floating fat particles. For ideas and recipes using *Mock Sour Cream,* see the chart showing how to use the Seven Survival Staples on pages 106 and 107.

¼ cup strained buttermilk or yogurt (1% or less fat, by weight)
1 cup cottage cheese (1% or less fat, by weight)
½ teaspoon lemon juice or vinegar, or more, to taste (if using buttermilk)

Pour the buttermilk or yogurt into a blender and add the cheese. Blend and stir as required to mix well. Add more buttermilk or yogurt, if necessary, to obtain a smooth consistency and desired thickness, and blend again. Blend in the lemon juice or vinegar, if using buttermilk.

Makes about 1 cup.

BERRY-APPLE COMPOTE

This recipe has special status as one of the Seven Survival Staples because it's an easy-to-make versatile dessert that can be prepared any time of year from two main ingredients— fresh apples plus a bag of frozen berries or cherries. Three versions are suggested in the recipe—each with individual flavor and somewhat different consistency—cherry-apple, strawberry-apple, and cranberry-apple. You can try still other kinds of berries for additional variety. Eat the compotes alone, or as a topping for a fresh or fresh- and frozen-fruit cup; or mix with yogurt (1% or less fat, by weight) or *Mock Sour*

Cream and use as a dessert or dessert topping. An elegant parfait can be made by alternating layers of the compote with the yogurt or *Mock Sour Cream,* ending with a garnish of crushed dry cereal. Use as a sweet topping for breakfast toast, or make into a party mold using plain unflavored gelatin. *Cranberry-Apple Compote* is excellent served with sliced chicken or turkey as a cold relish. The compotes may be frozen, but may become a little runny after thawing. To restore original consistency, reheat and again thicken with cornstarch as directed in the recipe.

    1½ cups water
    ¾ cup frozen apple juice concentrate
    1 teaspoon vanilla extract
 ½ to 1 teaspoon lemon extract, to taste
    1 12-ounce bag of frozen cherries, strawberries, or
      cranberries (you may also use fresh cranberries)
 3–4 apples, peeled and sliced
1½ to 2 tablespoons cornstarch, or more, if you prefer a thicker
      compote

Combine the liquid ingredients in a saucepan and bring to a boil. Add cherries, strawberries, or cranberries, and apples, and again return to a boil. Reduce heat and let simmer, uncovered, for 10–15 minutes. Make a paste of the cornstarch with 2 tablespoons of water and stir into the saucepan. Stir constantly until thickened. Let cool, then place in the refrigerator to chill.

Makes about 5 cups.

FROZEN BANANAS

If you think we've stretched the point in including frozen bananas in our list of survival staples, wait until you've tasted some of the concoctions that can be made with them. Assuming you're like most of us and have a bit of a sweet tooth, you'll certainly agree that frozen bananas should be one of the select group of survival staples which together can keep you well-nourished and happy, with minimal effort.

For the most part, frozen bananas perform their special magic by providing a smooth, bland, sweet base for blender-made shakes called "smoothies," or for soft and delectable "ice cream," made in a food processor. Sorry about the need for having these appliances to make these sweet snacks. But truly, if you use a blender and food processor for nothing else, they're worth having just to make these treats.

Recipes for making smoothies and the "ice cream" follow. There's also a recipe for making a frozen carob-covered banana-on-a-stick that was inspired by the frozen chocolate-covered bananas that used to be so popular.

Select ripe bananas for freezing. Peel them, cut away any bruised areas, and place them in a plastic bag. Don't overlap the bananas, as they may be difficult to separate when frozen if they're stuck together.

SUGGESTIONS FOR DINNER MENUS

In the dinner menu suggestions that follow, starred recipes are dishes made using Survival Staples as ingredients. The numbers in parentheses after the recipe names indicate the pages on which the recipes are located. Accompany your dinner meals, when appropriate, with lots of good whole-grain bread. If you wish to add more courses, easily prepared foods such as baked potatoes, baked yams or sweet potatoes, fresh or frozen corn-on-the-cob, or steamed green vegetables are possibilities to consider for almost any meal. Use lots of vegetables in your green salads, including plenty of dark green lettuce.

There are 16 menu plans in all. Feel free to use them in whole or in part or in any combination, so long as you adhere to the Pritikin diet guidelines (page 89). The possibilities for other dinner menu combinations using the Seven Survival Staples and other recipes in this book are seemingly endless, and you will certainly develop your own favorite menus in time.

1

Chicken Ratatouille* (148) over hot *Cooked Brown Rice (116)*
Baked Yam
Tossed Green Salad with *Creamy Artichoke Dressing* (192)*
Parfait of *Berry-Apple Compote (122)* and *Mock Sour Cream (121)*
in alternating layers, ending with crushed dry-cereal garnish

2

Spaghetti Sauce with Tomato-Veggie Stew* (164) over hot Whole-
Wheat Pasta
Tossed Green Salad with *Creamy French Dressing (193)*
Smoothie* (214)

3

Oven Bean Casserole* (139)
Baked Potato with *Mock Sour Cream (121)* topping
Steamed Corn-on-the-Cob or *Corn Bread (204)*
Tossed Green Salad with *Vinaigrette Dressing (194)*
Berry-Apple Compote (122) over Fresh Fruit Cup

4

Simmered *Creole-Style Fish (161)* served over hot *Cooked Brown
Rice (116)*
Steamed Artichoke with *Mustard-Yogurt Topping (194)*
Tossed Green Salad with *Creamy French Dressing (193)*
Pineapple "Ice Cream"* (213)

5

Chicken Tacos* (151)
Assorted Raw Vegetable Garnishes

Hot *Cooked Dried Beans (117)* topped with *Tomato-Veggie Stew (120)*
Berry-Apple Compote Meringue (208)*

6

Salmon-Rice Patties (138)*
Boiled New Potatoes with topping of *Mock Sour Cream (121)* or
Yogurt (1% or less fat, by weight)
Steamed Green Beans and Carrot Rounds
Lettuce with *Thousand Island Dressing* (193)*
Smoothie (214)*

7

Bean Enchiladas (140)*
Spanish Rice (133)* or hot *Cooked Brown Rice (116)*
Corn Kernels topped with *Tomato-Veggie Stew (120)*
Tossed Green Salad with *Vinaigrette Dressing (194)*
Fresh Fruit

8

Oven-Breaded Fish (160) with *Creole Sauce (161)*
Boiled or Baked Potato with topping of *Mock Sour Cream (121)* or
Yogurt (1% or less fat, by weight)
Steamed Greens
Sliced Tomatoes on bed of Lettuce
Carrot-Yam Cake (210)

9

Chicken Curry (149)* with Assorted Garnishes
Indian Rice (135)* or hot *Cooked Brown Rice (116)*
Cucumbers with Yogurt (180)
Orange "Ice Cream" (213)*

10

Pita Pizzas (166)
Whole-Wheat Spaghetti topped with *Tomato-Veggie Stew (120)*

Mixed Green Salad with *Creamy French Dressing (193)*
Berry-Apple Compote (122) over Fresh- and Frozen-Fruit Cup

11

Chili* (146) served over hot *Cooked Brown Rice (116)*
Steamed Broccoli Spears
Tossed Green Salad with *Vinaigrette Dressing (194)*
Smoothie* (214)

12

Onion Dip* (195) with Raw Vegetable Relishes
Sliced Simmered Chicken (118) or Sliced Breast of Turkey
Mashed Potatoes (189)
Mushroom Cream Sauce (166) or *Onion Gravy (190)*
Cranberry-Apple Compote* (Berry-Apple Compote, page *122)*
Steamed Brussels Sprouts
Pumpkin "Ice Cream"* (213)

13

Minestrone* (177)
Tropical Tuna Salad* (184)
Berry-Apple Compote (122) gelatinized and served in a mold
Lettuce with *Thousand Island Dressing* (193)*
Date Cake (209)

14

Chicken Crêpes with White Sauce* (154) with Sliced Orange
Garnish
Hawaiian Rice* (134) or hot *Cooked Brown Rice (116)*
Steamed Asparagus Spears
Tossed Green Salad with *Creamy French Dressing (193)*
Baked Apple Crumb (212)

15

Hummus Dip* (197) with Raw Vegetable Relishes
"Little Beef Burgers" (172) on Whole-Wheat Bread or Roll

Burger Sauce (172)
Lettuce, Tomato Slices, Onion Slices
"French Fries" (190)
Carob "Ice Cream" * (213)*

IMPORTANT POINTS ABOUT THE RECIPES

Before the recipes, a few general instructions concerning in-gredients and procedures:

RECIPE INGREDIENTS

- *Vegetable or fruit size:* When size is not specified, average size is intended. If small- or large-sized vegetables or fruits are to be used, size is specified.

- *Sodium content:* To reduce sodium content of recipes, use available brands of salt-reduced or no-salt-added condi-ments (such as soy sauce and Dijon-style mustard) to re-place normally high-sodium-content condiments. If you wish to further reduce sodium content, use other salt-restricted ingredients whenever possible.

- *Dairy products:* Yogurt and cottage cheese with fat content of 1% or less, by weight, are specified. Lowfat cottage cheese that has been rinsed in a strainer until rinse water runs clear may be used occasionally when the specified kind is unavailable. Purchase brands of buttermilk with lowest fat content, and before using, pour contents of entire con-tainer through a strainer to remove fat particles large enough to be strained out. (The recipes specify "strained buttermilk.") Nonfat milk is specified in general, except occasionally when the creamier quality of canned evaporated skim milk is desirable. Evaporated skim milk, however, has more than twice the protein (and caloric) content of nonfat milk, so if you want to take larger serving portions of a dish calling for evaporated skim milk, you may wish to substitute nonfat milk in the recipe.

- *Frozen apple juice concentrate:* This is the ingredient most often called for as a recipe sweetener. It should be measured out in the thawed state; so, for convenience, keep a can on your refrigerator door, defrosted.

- *Pepper:* When the addition of pepper to a recipe is desirable, cayenne pepper has been specified, as black pepper (and white pepper, a derivative) are suspected carcinogens.

- *Bread crumbs:* Fine whole-wheat bread crumbs made from an acceptable bread are an ingredient in some recipes. To make them, use an electric blender or food processor.

- *Stock:* Defatted chicken stock is specified as an ingredient in certain recipes because of its flavor-enhancing quality. Vegetable stock can be used as a substitute, if you like. Save the liquid left over after steaming vegetables for this purpose, or cook up a vegetable stock. (To a large soup pot filled with boiling water add clean vegetable scraps; a couple of large onions, quartered, a few halved leeks and celery stalks; a small handful of garlic cloves, a few parsley sprigs, and a bay leaf, and let cook for 1 hour or more. Strain the stock and it's ready for use. Store in freezer in convenient-sized containers.)

RECIPE PROCEDURES

- *Special cooking techniques:* To replace conventional sautée-ing in oils, we have developed two sautéeing procedures: 1) liquid sautéeing, in which the ingredients are cooked in a skillet, stirring as needed, in a small amount of fat-free liquid, such as defatted chicken stock, vegetable stock, or just water; and 2) dry-sautéeing, in which the ingredients are placed directly on the heated skillet surface, and cooked over low heat for a few minutes while stirring constantly to prevent scorching. You'll find the two methods very simple and the results most satisfactory.

- *Modifying recipe yield or ingredients:* Don't hesitate to in-dividualize the recipes to suit your needs and preferences. For instance, you may wish to double or halve the recipe size or to modify the seasoning. Just make sure that what-ever changes you make don't conflict with the nutritional guidelines (pages 89–90 and 97–102).

- *Preheating oven:* With some recipes, it's critically impor-tant that the food be set into a preheated oven. When an oven temperature is given, wait before putting it in until the oven has reached the specified temperature.

- *Rinsing of ingredients:* Some preliminary preparation of produce, poultry, rice, legumes, and other ingredients is necessary. Dried beans and peas (legumes) may need some sorting through. Both legumes and brown rice should be rinsed before cooking. Wash fruits and vegetables thor-oughly, and peel any waxed fruits or vegetables, as well as vegetables with coarse skins, such as rutabagas or turnips. Fresh or frozen fish and poultry should be rinsed in cold water, then patted dry with paper towels.

● *Useful equipment:* Besides standard kitchen equipment, you'll need nonstick baking sheets and one or more nonstick skillets, and a steamer basket for steaming foods. A blender and a food processor, two handy electric appliances, will reduce the time and labor involved in the chopping of onions and other vegetables, making bread crumbs, puréeing foods, and other procedures.

RECIPES

Recipes using one or more of the survival staples as ingredients have their titles italicized and are followed by an asterisk; within these recipes, the survival staple ingredients also appear in italics. A chart listing all the recipes using the survival staples appears on pages 104–108. Recipes for the survival staples themselves are on pages 115–124.

HOT RICE DISHES

CHINESE "FRIED" RICE *

This rice dish can be a meal all by itself. Be sure to add the pea pods and bean sprouts near the end of the cooking period, so their crunchy texture is retained.

      1 onion, chopped
      1 cup chopped celery
      2 cloves garlic, finely chopped
      2 egg whites, lightly beaten
      2 cups sliced mushrooms
      1 8-ounce can sliced bamboo shoots, drained
    1½ tablespoons soy sauce
    1–2 cups chopped *simmered chicken* (optional)
      1 6-ounce package frozen pea pods, or 1 cup fresh pea pods
      4 cups fresh bean sprouts
      2 cups *cooked brown rice*

Combine the onion, celery, and garlic in a bowl. In a large skillet or wok over low heat, dry-sauté about ½ cup of the vegetable mixture, stirring constantly for about 2 minutes to partially tenderize the vegetables. Pour the egg whites on top of the vegetables in the skillet to coagulate them. When they have turned white, add the rest of the vegetables in the bowl, and stir and sauté for another few minutes until the vegetables are tenderized. Add the mushrooms, bamboo shoots, soy sauce, and chicken, and stir and cook another few minutes. Mix in the pea pods and bean sprouts and stir and cook about 2 minutes. Stir in the rice and heat through for just a few minutes.

Makes about 9 or 10 cups.

SPANISH RICE *

1 cup chopped onions
1 cup chopped celery
¾ cup chopped green pepper
⅔ cup canned diced chiles
1 cup canned tomato sauce
2 tablespoons canned tomato paste
1 tablespoon chile con carne seasoning or other Mexican
   seasoning blend
1 teaspoon cumin
2 cups *cooked brown rice*

Heat a large skillet and dry-sauté the onions, celery, and green pepper over low heat for about 5 minutes, stirring constantly. Add the chiles, tomato products, and seasoning, and mix well. Stir in the rice, and heat through for a few minutes, stirring constantly to prevent sticking.

Makes about 4 cups.

MEXICAN RICE *

1 cup defatted *chicken stock* or vegetable stock, or water
2 tomatoes, diced
⅔ cup diced carrots
½ cup chopped celery
½ cup sliced mushrooms
¼ cup minced parsley
2 garlic cloves, finely chopped
1 tablespoon dried onion flakes
1½ teaspoons marjoram
   Dash cayenne pepper
2 cups *cooked brown rice*

Bring the stock or water to a boil in a large skillet. Add all the ingredients, except the rice, lower heat, and cook for about 10 minutes, stirring occasionally. Stir in the rice, mixing lightly, and heat through for a few minutes. Serve with bottled hot sauce on the side.

Makes 4 cups.

HAWAIIAN RICE *

 1 cup chopped onions
 1 cup chopped celery
 ½ cup chopped green onions
 ⅓ cup raisins
 1 teaspoon grated fresh ginger
 1 8-ounce can crushed pineapple in own juices
 1 8-ounce can pineapple chunks in own juices
 1 8-ounce can water chestnuts, drained and sliced
 1 tablespoon onion powder
 ½ tablespoon soy sauce
 1 teaspoon vinegar
 2 cups *cooked brown rice*

Heat a large skillet and dry-sauté the onions, celery, green onions, raisins, and ginger over low heat for about 5 minutes, stirring constantly. Drain both cans of pineapple and add the juices to the skillet. Continue cooking for a few minutes until most of the liquid evaporates. Add the pineapple and water chestnuts, sprinkle on the onion powder, and stir in the soy sauce and vinegar. Mix lightly to combine flavors. Stir in the rice, and heat through for a few minutes, stirring constantly to prevent sticking.

Makes about 5 cups.

INDIAN RICE *

1 cup chopped onions
1 cup chopped celery
½ cup orange juice
2 tablespoons chopped mint leaves
1 tablespoon onion powder
1 teaspoon curry powder
2 cups *cooked brown rice*
⅔ cup frozen green peas (optional)

Heat a large skillet and dry-sauté the onions and celery over low heat for about 3–5 minutes, stirring constantly. Add the orange juice and continue cooking and stirring for a few minutes until most of the liquid is evaporated. Stir in the mint leaves, sprinkle on the onion powder and curry powder, and mix lightly to combine flavors. Stir in the rice, and heat through for a few minutes, stirring constantly to prevent sticking. If adding green peas, rinse the frozen peas in a strainer under cold water to separate them, drain well, and add to the skillet after adding the rice.

Makes 5 cups.

CONFETTI RICE *

1 onion, chopped
1 green pepper, chopped
2 cups frozen corn kernels
1 4-ounce jar sliced pimiento, chopped
1 teaspoon oregano
½ teaspoon paprika
½ tablespoon soy sauce
1 cup frozen green peas
2 cups *cooked brown rice*

In a large skillet, dry-sauté the onion and green pepper over low heat, stirring constantly, until the vegetables are tender-crisp (about 5 minutes). Add the corn, pimiento, and season-ings, and continue cooking for 2–3 minutes, stirring as needed. Stir in the green peas and rice, and heat thoroughly for about 5 minutes, stirring occasionally as required.

Makes 6 cups.

RICE-BULGUR PILAF*

In this version of a traditional Middle Eastern recipe, bulgur wheat and garbanzo beans team up with rice and vegetables for a different kind of grain dish.

    1 cup water plus 1 teaspoon soy sauce
    1 teaspoon onion powder
    ½ cup raw bulgur wheat
    1 cup chopped onions
    1 cup chopped celery
    2 cloves garlic, finely minced
    2 tablespoons chopped mint leaves
    1 small tomato, chopped
    1 tablespoon soy sauce
    1 10-ounce package frozen peas and carrots
    1 cup *cooked garbanzo beans* (or 1 15-ounce can garbanzos),
       drained
    2 cups *cooked brown rice*

Bring the water and soy sauce and the onion powder to a boil in a small saucepan. Stir in the bulgur wheat, reduce heat to low, cover, and let cook for about 5 minutes. Turn off heat and let sit, covered, 15 minutes or longer. While bulgur wheat is sitting, place the onions, celery, garlic, and half the mint in a large skillet over low heat, and dry-sauté the vegetables for about 5 minutes or until they are tenderized, stirring fre-quently. Add the chopped tomato, soy sauce, and the rest of the mint leaves, and continue cooking and stirring for another few minutes. Place the peas and carrots in a colander and pour hot water over them for a minute or two. Add the peas, carrots, and garbanzo beans to the skillet, and cook and stir for another minute or two. Stir in the rice and the bulgur, and heat through for a few minutes.

Makes 8 cups.

Cooked brown rice is a key ingredient in the two fish-rice dishes that follow. They offer very different ways of using your cooked rice.

TUNA-RICE BAKE *

1   6½ ounce can tuna (packed in water), drained and flaked
3   cups *cooked brown rice*
1   cup frozen corn kernels
1   cup chopped green pepper
1   cup chopped celery
1   large onion, chopped
1   2-ounce jar sliced pimientos
3   egg whites
¼   cup potato flour (or, if preferred, rice or wheat flour)
    Sprinkling of fine whole-wheat bread crumbs (from acceptable bread)

Sauce (optional): *Tomato-Veggie Stew*

Combine the tuna, rice, corn, chopped vegetables, pimientos, and egg whites in a large bowl. Stir in the potato flour. Transfer to a 7" × 11" nonstick or Pyrex baking dish, spreading the mixture evenly over the dish or mounding it in loaf fashion, as preferred. Top with a sprinkling of bread crumbs. Place in a 350° oven and bake uncovered for about 50–60 minutes, or until sides and top look done. Remove from oven and let cool 15 minutes or longer, before cutting into servings. Serve topped with hot *Tomato-Veggie Stew,* if desired.

Makes 8 servings.

SALMON-RICE PATTIES *

1 15½ ounce can pink or red salmon
1 small onion, coarsely chopped
2 cups *cooked brown rice*
2 egg whites
½ tablespoon dillweed
½ tablespoon onion powder
½ teaspoon tarragon
½ cup potato flour or, if preferred, rice or wheat flour

Drain the salmon, and remove the skin and bones. Place salmon in a bowl. Put the other ingredients, except the potato flour, in a food processor or blender, and process for a few minutes to chop rice and onions. Transfer processed contents to the bowl and mix in the potato flour. Form into patties and arrange them on a nonstick baking sheet. Bake, uncovered, in a 450° oven for 20 minutes. Serve with *Mustard-Yogurt Topping* (page 194).

Makes 12 patties.

HOT BEAN DISHES

In the hot bean dishes that follow, you can season the recipes to your taste by increasing or decreasing the amount of chiles or chile seasoning used. When working with chilies, especially the hotter varieties, remember to mince finely, since a little goes a long way; always remove seeds, membranes, and stems; and—in order to avoid possible skin irritation—do not touch any part of your face until you've washed your hands after handling them.

BARREGO BEANS *

  2 cups chopped onions
  2 cups chopped celery
  ½ seeded jalapeño chile, finely chopped
  2 cups *cooked pinto beans*, drained
  1 28-ounce can whole tomatoes, undrained, coarsely chopped

Place the onions and celery in a wide-bottomed pot or skillet and dry-sauté, stirring constantly for about 10 minutes. Stir in the chile, and continue to dry-sauté and stir for another 5 minutes. Mix in the beans, and let heat through for a few minutes, stirring occasionally. Pour over the tomatoes and heat through.

Makes 6 cups.

BEAN CASSEROLES *

Choose one of two versions. Version I is quicker if you have on hand the two survival staples required, since it merely combines them and a few seasonings. Version II requires some vegetable cutting, but can also be rapidly put together to make a delicious hot dish. If you have leftovers from either version, recycle them as *tacos, tostadas,* or *burritos,* assembling the principal ingredients—corn tortillas, raw vegetables, and beans—in the manner described on page 143.

Version 1
    3 cups *cooked pinto beans, or other beans of choice,* drained
    2½ cups *Tomato-Veggie Stew*
    ½ cup water
    1½ tablespoons chile powder
    1 teaspoon cumin

Combine ingredients and place in a baking dish. Bake covered in a 350° oven for about 45 minutes, removing the cover after about 30 minutes.

Makes 4–6 servings.

Version 2
    3 cups *cooked pinto beans, or other beans of choice,* drained
    1 large red onion, chopped
    1 green pepper, chopped
    1 28-ounce can crushed tomatoes
    1 tablespoon curry powder
    1 tablespoon cornstarch

Combine ingredients and place in a baking dish. Bake covered in a 400° oven for about an hour, removing cover after about 30 minutes.

Makes 4–6 servings.

BEAN ENCHILADAS *

If you're not going to be serving all the enchiladas at once, it's a good idea to freeze the ones you won't be eating for a while *before* baking them. They reheat best from the frozen state if they haven't been baked previously. Place the unbaked enchiladas in a container for freezing and pour a little sauce over them, then freeze; or, if you wish, you can make "bean rolls," wrapping enchiladas individually in aluminum foil, without adding sauce. The "bean rolls" (or "burritos") may be reheated right in the foil in an oven for snacks or lunches. If making "bean rolls," be sure to tuck in the ends of the corn tortillas when filling the enchiladas, to seal them securely.

> 3 cups *cooked pinto beans, or other beans of choice,* drained
> 1 large onion, chopped
> ½ cup canned green chile salsa
> ¼ cup canned diced chiles
> 1 tablespoon chile con carne seasoning blend or other Mexican seasoning blend
> 1 teaspoon each: onion powder, garlic powder, and cumin
> 12 corn tortillas

Sauce:
> 1 15-ounce can tomato sauce, mixed with 1 tablespoon chile powder,
> *or* 2 cups *Tomato-Veggie Stew,* blended in blender with 1 tablespoon chile powder

Mash the beans and set them aside. In a small skillet, sauté the onions together with the seasonings until the onions are soft. Combine the beans and seasoned onions, mixing well. Separate, then heat tortillas in a 350° oven until softened. Remove from oven and fill each with some of the mashed bean mixture, and roll up. Place seam-side down in a nonstick baking pan, taking care not to overlap, and cover each with a little sauce. Bake uncovered in a 350° oven for 10–15 minutes.

Makes 12 enchiladas.

REFRIED BEANS

In this recipe, the dried beans are cooked *together* with the other ingredients. *Refried Beans* are excellent for making *tacos, tostadas,* and *burritos,* using the method of assembling the beans, corn tortillas, and raw vegetables described on page 143. To use as a dip, simply thin the *Refried Beans* with additional canned green chile salsa.

2 cups uncooked dried pinto beans, washed and picked over
1 large onion, chopped
2 stalks celery, chopped
1 large carrot, chopped
3 cups water
1 cup canned tomato sauce
½ cup canned green chile salsa
1½ tablespoons chile con carne seasoning or other Mexican seasoning blend
1 tablespoon soy sauce
1 tablespoon onion powder
½ tablespoon garlic powder

Place all of the ingredients in a large pot. Bring to a boil, turn heat to very low, and simmer, covered, for about 2 hours, or until beans are soft, stirring occasionally as required. Mash with a hand masher, or place in a blender or food processor to mash. Avoid overprocessing.

Makes 5½ cups.

TACOS, TOSTADAS, AND BURRITOS *

Combine seasoned *cooked beans* and corn tortillas (never flour tortillas; they contain lard) to make your choice of these tasty Mexican dishes. You can use plain cooked pinto or red beans, mashed and seasoned with onion and garlic powders, and canned green chile salsa, to taste; or leftover beans from such recipes as *Bean Casseroles* (page 140) or *Refried Beans* (page 141).

TACO AND TOSTADA *

Reheat bean mixture. While beans are heating, prepare vegetable garnishes to go over the beans: shred some lettuce and place it in a small serving bowl; slice or dice tomatoes and place in another bowl; in a third bowl, combine some chopped green onion, chopped green pepper, and a little crumbly dry cottage cheese (under 1% fat, by weight), if desired.

To make a *taco,* heat a corn tortilla in a hot oven until it is hot but still pliable. Place a few tablespoons of hot beans in the center, fold in half, then stuff in some of each of the raw vegetable garnishes. Add a few drops of bottled hot sauce or taco sauce. Eat out of hand, sandwich-style.

To make a *tostada,* heat a corn tortilla in a hot oven until it is lightly browned and rather crisp. Pile a few tablespoons of hot beans in the center, flatten them out with a spoon towards the edges, and pile on raw vegetables and condiments as for the *taco,* above. Eat out of hand like an open-faced sandwich.

BURRITO *

Heat a corn tortilla in a hot oven until it is hot but still pliable. Place hot beans in the center and roll up, tucking in the ends to seal securely. Accompany with a mixed green salad. If you wish, make bean rolls for the freezer for future use. Wrap each bean roll individually in aluminum foil to be reheated later in the foil in an oven for quick snacks or take-out lunches.

HUEVOS RANCHEROS *

In this interpretation of Mexican "ranch eggs," cooked beans, "fried" egg whites, zesty seasonings, and corn tortillas are combined to make an appetizing brunch or light supper dish.

> 1 cup chopped onion
> ½ cup chopped pepper
> 2 cloves garlic, finely chopped
> 1 7-ounce can green chile salsa
> 1½ cups *cooked pinto beans,* drained
> 4 egg whites
> 4 corn tortillas

Garnish: paprika and chopped green onions

In a large nonstick skillet, dry-sauté the onions, green pepper, and garlic over low heat for about 5 minutes, until tenderized. Add the green chile salsa and continue cooking for a few minutes. Mash the beans a little, then stir them into the skillet mixture and continue to cook for a few minutes. Separate the bean-mixture into four mounds on the skillet and make a depression in each mound. Drop one egg white into each depression, cover, and let cook for about 5 minutes to coagulate egg whites. (Some of the egg white may flow over the depression; if you wish, scoop it back onto the beans.) Place the tortillas in a hot oven and let them heat until they are no longer soft and have browned lightly. Place a bean-egg mound on top of each of the four tortillas. Garnish the egg white with a sprinkling of paprika and chopped green onions. Serve with bottled hot sauce on the side.

Makes 4 servings.

PASTA E FAGIOLI *

This dish is meant to be served hot; but eaten cold, it tastes like a delicious pasta salad. So leftovers could go into your lunchbox.

½ cup defatted *chicken stock,* vegetable stock, or water
2 large onions, finely chopped
2 carrots, finely chopped
3 cloves garlic, minced or crushed
1 cup chopped parsley, divided
2 tablespoons basil
1 teaspoon oregano
3 large tomatoes, peeled and chopped
3 cups cooked whole-wheat pasta (cooked *al dente;* use elbow macaroni or corkscrew pasta, or a combination of the two)
¼ cup grated Sap Sago cheese
5 cups *cooked kidney beans,* drained

Heat the stock to a boil in a large pot and add the onions, carrots, garlic, ¾ cup of the parsley, basil, and oregano. Stir-fry the mixture over medium heat for about 6–8 minutes. Stir in the tomatoes; then cover and simmer over low heat for 8–10 minutes. Add the beans, mix well, and simmer another 20 minutes, stirring occasionally. Gently mix in the cooked pasta and heat thoroughly. Sprinkle the remaining parsley and the cheese over the top. If a spicy flavor is desired, serve a bottled hot sauce on the side.

Makes 8 servings.

BEAN-BULGUR COMBO *

This dish has so many virtues—it's flavorful, filling, colorful, and quickly assembled. In the years our sons were growing up, when the reply to the question "What's there to eat, Mom?" drew an unsatisfactory response, it was their favorite do-it-yourself dish to appease growling stomachs.

3 cups water plus 1½ teaspoons soy sauce
1½ teaspoons onion powder
1½ cups raw bulgur wheat

> 1 large onion, chopped
> 2 cloves garlic, finely chopped
> ¾ cup chopped green onions
> 1 7-ounce can green chile salsa
> 1 teaspoon chile powder
> 1 16-ounce can diced tomatoes, undrained
> 2 cups *cooked kidney, pinto, or red beans,* drained

Bring the water and soy sauce and the onion powder to a boil in a saucepan. Stir in the bulgur wheat, reduce heat to low, cover, and let cook for about 5 minutes. Turn off heat and let sit, covered, 15 minutes or longer. In a skillet, place the onions, garlic, and green onions, and dry-sauté over medium heat for about 5 minutes, stirring frequently. Add the green chile salsa and chile powder and cook and stir for another few minutes. Stir in the tomatoes and beans, and continue to cook and stir occasionally for another few minutes. Stir in the bulgur wheat and heat through briefly.

Makes 7 cups.

CHILI *

> ½ pound very lean beef (such as flank steak), ground
> 1 onion, chopped
> 1 green pepper, chopped
> 2 cloves garlic, finely chopped
> 2 cups *cooked kidney or pinto beans,* undrained
> 1 28-ounce can tomatoes, undrained, coarsely chopped
> 1 15-ounce can tomato sauce
> ¼ cup tomato paste, mixed with ¼ cup water
> 3 tablespoons chile con carne seasoning
> 1½ teaspoons dry mustard
> ½ teaspoon soy sauce

In a large skillet, brown the ground beef. Add the remaining ingredients. Simmer, covered, for ½ hour, stirring occasionally. Remove cover, and continue to simmer another ½ hour, stirring as required. Serve with hot cooked brown rice, or whole-wheat pasta.

Makes 4 servings.

Lentils are related to beans and are a good substitute for them. They have an advantage in cooking much more quickly (about 35 minutes), without a presoaking period. The two recipes that follow use lentils in very different ways. *Spicy Mexican Lentils* are prepared as a stew, perfect over cooked brown rice or potatoes, or combined with corn tortillas to make *tacos* or *tostadas* (see page 143). Then, if you like, you can use the leftover lentil mixture to make *Lentil Patties,* following the instructions for the easy recipe variation on page 148.

SPICY MEXICAN LENTILS

1½ cups lentils
1 onion, chopped
5 cloves garlic, minced or crushed
½ cup chopped fresh cilantro (Mexican or Chinese parsley); *or,* if preferred, use regular parsley
½ fresh green chile, seeded and minced; *or* 1 teaspoon chile powder
1½ teaspoons ground cumin
1 teaspoon ground coriander
1 7-ounce can green chile salsa
2 cups canned tomato sauce
2 cups water

Place all the ingredients in a pot. Bring to a boil, then reduce heat to moderate, cover, and cook until the lentils are tender (about 30–40 minutes), stirring frequently.

Makes 6 cups.

Variation: LENTIL PATTIES *

2½ cups *Spicy Mexican Lentils*
1½ cups *cooked brown rice*
 2 egg whites
 ½ cup potato flour (or, if preferred, rice or wheat flour)

Place the lentil mixture in a bowl. Put the rice, egg whites, and potato flour in a blender and blend for a few minutes to chop the rice. Transfer the blender mixture to the bowl and mix well. Form into patties, place on a nonstick baking sheet, and bake in a 400° oven for 25 minutes. Place under the broiler for a minute or two for additional light browning, if desired.

Makes 9 patties.

HOT CHICKEN DISHES

CHICKEN RATATOUILLE *

This delicious chicken dish is made by combining two survival staples—*simmered chicken* and *Tomato-Veggie Stew*. Since *Tomato-Veggie Stew* is a first cousin to traditional *ratatouille,* it's a logical union.

3½ cups *Tomato-Veggie Stew*
1½ cups *simmered chicken,* cut into chunks

Combine the stew and chicken and place in an oven casserole. Heat, uncovered, in a 350° oven for 15–20 minutes. Serve over hot cooked brown rice. (If desired, the rice may be heated at the same time in a separate ovenproof dish, closely covered to avoid drying it out and to permit it to steam.)

Makes 3 servings.

CHICKEN CURRY *

2½ cups defatted *chicken stock*
 ½ cup finely chopped onions
 1 stalk celery with leaves, finely chopped
 2 large cloves garlic, finely chopped
 1 large apple, peeled and coarsely grated
1½ tablespoons finely chopped ginger
1½ tablespoons curry powder
 2 tablespoons canned tomato paste
 ½ cup white vermouth
1½ tablespoons frozen apple juice concentrate
   Juice of 1 lime
1½ tablespoons cornstarch
1½ cups diced *simmered chicken*
   Assorted garnishes as suggested below

Place ½ cup of the chicken stock in a large pot. Add the onions, celery, garlic, apple, and ginger; sauté over medium heat, stirring constantly, until the liquid has almost evaporated. Stir in the spices and tomato paste. Add the remaining chicken stock and bring to a boil, then cover, turn down the heat, and simmer for 20 minutes.

Make a smooth mixture of the vermouth, apple juice concentrate, lime juice, and cornstarch. Add this mixture to the simmering sauce and continue simmering for a few minutes until slightly thickened. Stir in the diced chicken just before serving; heat thoroughly. Serve over hot brown rice with assorted garnishes. Suggested garnishes are a few raisins, chopped green onions, sliced bananas, and *Cucumbers with Yogurt* (page 180).

Makes 3 servings.

CHICKEN À LA KING *

This recipe may also be used to make *tuna à la king* by substituting 2 cups chunks of canned white-meat tuna (packed in water) for the chicken. Tuna should be added only 1 or 2 minutes before removing the pot from the stove. Also, replace the Fines Herbes with ½ teaspoon tarragon, a better spice for the tuna.

    ½ pound mushrooms, sliced
    1 small onion, chopped
    1 stalk celery, chopped
    2 cloves garlic, finely chopped
    2 cups defatted *chicken stock*
    1½ cups canned evaporated skim milk
    2 tablespoons cornstarch
    ¼ cup dry sherry
    1 cup frozen green peas, thawed
    1 2-ounce jar diced pimientos
    1 tablespoon chopped parsley
    1 teaspoon curry powder
    ½ teaspoon spice blend, such as Spice Islands Fines Herbes
    ½ teaspoon Tabasco
    1½ cups *simmered chicken*, cut into chunks

In a skillet, sauté the mushrooms, onions, celery, and garlic in a few tablespoons of water over medium heat until tender. Set aside. Prepare a double boiler (you can fit a stainless steel bowl over a pot of boiling water) and place the chicken stock and milk in the bowl. Heat the liquids until they are very hot and start to bubble. Blend the cornstarch with the sherry to make a paste, and stir into the very hot stock/milk mixture. Continue to stir until the mixture thickens. Add the green peas, sautéed vegetables, and other ingredients. Stir gently and cook for 5 to 10 minutes until mixture is heated through. Serve over hot brown rice, whole-wheat pasta, baked potato, or toasted whole-wheat English muffins.

Makes 4 servings.

CHICKEN TACOS *

Filling:
- ¼ cup defatted *chicken stock*
- 1 cup finely chopped onions
- ¾ cup finely chopped green or red bell pepper
- ¼ cup chopped fresh cilantro (Mexican or Chinese parsley)
- 1 4-ounce can diced green chiles
- 2 cups diced *simmered chicken*
- 1½ cups *cooked brown rice*
- 2 teaspoons soy sauce
- 1½ teaspoons basil
- 1 teaspoon garlic powder
- Dash cayenne pepper

- 12 corn tortillas

Raw Vegetable Garnishes: shredded lettuce, diced tomatoes, and chopped green onions

In a skillet, bring the stock to a boil and add the onions and bell pepper. Sauté the vegetables over medium heat until softened, for about 5–7 minutes. Add the cilantro, chiles, chicken, rice, and seasonings; stir well, cover, and cook over low heat for 4–5 minutes, or until thoroughly heated. Heat the tortillas, a few at a time, in a hot oven until they are hot but still pliable. Spoon about ⅓ cup of the chicken-rice mixture into each warmed tortilla, add raw vegetable garnishes, fold tortilla in half, and eat sandwich-style. A dollop of yogurt (1% or less fat, by weight), a few drops of bottled hot sauce or Picante sauce, and a little chopped fresh cilantro may be used as additional garnishes for extra flavor.

Makes 12 tacos.

CHICKEN ENCHILADAS *

Use the filling for *Chicken Tacos* (page 151) to make the filling for these delicious enchiladas. The sauce is simple to make.

    1 recipe *Chicken Tacos* filling
  12 corn tortillas

Sauce:
    1 15-ounce can tomato sauce, mixed with 1 tablespoon chile powder, or 2 cups *Tomato-Veggie Stew,* blended in blender with 1 tablespoon chile powder

Spread a thin layer of the sauce in a 10″ × 14″ nonstick baking pan. In a hot oven, heat tortillas, a few at a time, for a minute or two, until hot but still pliable. Remove and fill while still hot with about ⅓ cup filling each. Roll tortilla and place seam-side down in the pan. Repeat procedure until all the tortillas are filled, taking care not to overlap them in the pan. Pour the sauce over the enchiladas. Bake uncovered at 350° for 30 minutes. Serve with *Mock Sour Cream* or yogurt (1% or less fat, by weight). Garnish with chopped fresh cilantro or green onions.

Makes 12 enchiladas.

CHINESE STIR-FRY VEGETABLES
WITH CHICKEN *

Although there are a large number of ingredients to prepare, once that is done, this is a very simple dish to cook. Just be sure to have all the vegetables cut and other ingredients measured and ready to use before you start cooking. That will enable you to process the ingredients rapidly so that the vegetables will still be crisp at the end of the cooking period.

1¾ cups defatted *chicken stock*
  2 cloves garlic, minced
  2 cups slant-cut celery
  1 large onion, coarsely chopped
  1 cup sliced mushrooms
  ½ cup sliced canned water chestnuts
  1 large red or green bell pepper, chopped (red is prettier)
  5 cups Napa cabbage, coarsely slant-cut
  1 medium tomato, diced
  2 cups broccoli florets
  2 cups bean sprouts
  2 cups snow peas
  1 cup chopped green onions
1½ cups diced *simmered chicken*
  1 8-ounce can crushed pineapple in own juices
  ¼ cup white wine
  1 tablespoon soy sauce
  1 teaspoon grated fresh ginger or 1½ teaspoons powdered
    ginger
  1 teaspoon Chinese-style hot mustard
  4 tablespoons cornstarch

In a wok, skillet, or large pot, bring ½ cup of the stock to a boil. Add the garlic, celery, and onion, and sauté over medium heat for about 4 minutes, stirring frequently. Add the mushrooms, water chestnuts, and bell pepper, and continue stirring and sautéeing for about 2 minutes. Add the Napa cabbage, tomato, and broccoli, and continue stirring and sautéeing for another 2 minutes. Add the rest of the stock, bean sprouts, snow peas, green onions, chicken, and pineapple, and stir and sauté for another few minutes. In a bowl, combine the wine, soy sauce, ginger, mustard, and cornstarch. Stir to dissolve the cornstarch, and add the mixture to the simmering vegetables and chicken. Continue stirring until the liquid thickens. Serve over hot cooked brown rice.

Makes 3–5 servings.

CHICKEN CRÊPES WITH WHITE SAUCE *

The delicately flavored sauce for these crêpes is made with whey powder, a nonfat dry-milk product available in health-food stores. You can use this same recipe to make crab crêpes, substituting about 10 ounces of cooked crab meat for the chicken.

Sauce:
   1 cup canned evaporated skim milk
   2 cups defatted *chicken stock* or vegetable stock
   ¼ cup whey powder
   2½ tablespoons cornstarch
   1 tablespoon dry white wine
   ½ cup diced red bell pepper or canned pimientos
   ⅛ teaspoon curry powder

Filling:
   ½ cup defatted *chicken stock* or vegetable stock
   1 tablespoon dry white wine
   2 cups finely chopped celery
   1½ cups finely chopped onions
   1 teaspoon spice blend, such as Spice Islands Bouquet Garni
   ¼ teaspoon curry powder
   2 cups diced *simmered chicken*

Crêpes:
   1½ cups nonfat milk
   ¾ cup strained buttermilk

1½ cups whole-wheat pastry flour
1 tablespoon baking powder
4 egg whites

Sauce: Pour the milk and 1 cup of the stock into a saucepan and heat to a simmer. In a bowl, stir together the whey powder, cornstarch, and remaining stock. Add the whey/cornstarch mixture to the simmering liquid and stir constantly until the sauce is smooth and thickened. Stir in the wine, red bell pepper, and curry powder. Remove from heat and set aside.

Filling: In a skillet, bring the stock and wine to a boil. Add the celery and onions and sauté over moderate heat until they are nearly tender. Stir in the curry powder, Bouquet Garni, and chicken. Set aside.

Crêpes: In a blender, pour the milks, flour, baking powder, and egg whites. Blend until very smooth. Bake the crêpes on a nonstick skillet or crêpe pan. To reduce the possibility of sticking, you may wish to dab a little oil on a paper towel (or Handi-Wipe), rinse towel in water and wring it out, then wipe over the skillet or crêpe pan surface whenever sticking is a problem, but do not add more oil to the towel. Place the pan over moderate heat. Pour about ½ cup of batter into the pan, spreading it around evenly, and brown one side. Turn the crêpe and lightly brown the other side. Remove any baked particles from the pan before adding new batter for the next crêpe.

Carefully remove each crêpe to a plate and fill with about ⅓ cup of filling. Tuck the corners in, if desired, and roll. Lay the filled crêpe seam-side down on a nonstick baking pan. Repeat this procedure until all the crêpes have been filled and arranged in the pan. Spoon some white sauce over the crêpes, cover, and bake at 375° for 15–20 minutes. Reheat the remaining white sauce and serve with the crêpes.

Makes approximately 12 filled crêpes and 3 cups sauce.

CHICKEN AND OKRA GUMBO *

This classic Creole dish has been adapted for Pritikin guidelines, but you'll still need to make a *roux,* the traditional browned-flour technique for thickening dishes. Make sure you brown the flour carefully, to avoid burning it. To make a fish and okra gumbo, just substitute 2 cups chunked, raw halibut or other firm-fleshed white fish, adding the fish 5–10 minutes before the end of the cooking time.

          2 onions, choppped
          1 green pepper, chopped
          2 cloves garlic, finely minced
         ½ cup chopped green onion bottoms
          4 cups defatted *chicken stock*
         ⅓ cup whole-wheat pastry flour
          1 28-ounce can whole tomatoes, undrained
         ½ tablespoon soy sauce (optional)
          1 tablespoon gumbo filé
     1½ teaspoons ground celery seed
         ½ teaspoon basil
         ½ teaspoon Tabasco
             Pinch of cayenne pepper
          3 cups sliced okra, fresh or frozen
          2 cups diced *simmered chicken*

Place the onions, green pepper, garlic, and green onions in a soup pot and dry-sauté over low heat for about 7 minutes, stirring frequently. Set pot aside. In a skillet, brown the flour over low heat, stirring constantly until flour is browned but not too dark. Add ½ cup of the stock (it should not be hot) and stir to make a paste with the flour. Quarter the tomatoes, and add to the soup pot together with the tomato liquid and the rest of the stock. Bring to a boil, turn down heat to a simmer, and slowly add the flour paste, stirring to blend well. Add the seasonings and cook slowly for 30 minutes, partially covered, stirring occasionally to prevent sticking. Sauté the okra in a skillet with a little water or broth from the cooking pot; cook about 5 minutes, or until somewhat dry and less slick. Add the okra and the diced chicken to the soup pot about 10 minutes before the end of the cooking time. Serve over hot cooked brown rice, with bottled hot sauce on the side.

Makes 6–8 servings (11 cups).

When you want a change from simmered-chicken recipes, the next easiest approach for preparing chicken dishes is to use raw boneless chicken breasts. Buy small ones (about 5 ounces for a half boned breast with skin on), so each serving is within Pritikin diet guidelines after skinning. Then proceed with one of the delicious chicken recipes that follow.

CHICKEN BREASTS AUX CHAMPIGNONS

1 cup fine whole-wheat bread crumbs (from acceptable bread— that is, whole-grain wheat bread without oil)
4 small boneless chicken breast halves, skinned
½ cup canned evaporated skim milk
2 cups sliced mushrooms
2 tablespoons diced shallots
½ cup dry white wine
1 teaspoon lemon juice
⅛ teaspoon thyme
⅛ teaspoon marjoram

Mushroom Cream Sauce (page 166)

Prepare the bread crumbs by processing bread in a food processor or blender. Pound the chicken breasts flat with a meat mallet. Dip each breast in the milk and then in the bread crumbs, covering well. Roll up each breast and arrange seam-side down in a nonstick baking pan, cover, and bake at 350° for 25 minutes.

Meanwhile, sauté the mushrooms and shallots in the wine and lemon juice, stirring in the seasonings as the vegetables cook. Uncover the chicken and spoon some of the sautéed vegetables over each chicken breast. Bake uncovered 10 minutes longer, or until the chicken is tender and brown. Just before serving, ladle *Mushroom Cream Sauce* over each chicken breast.

Makes 4 servings.

CHICKEN AND POTATOES
IN MUSHROOM-TOMATO SAUCE

        5 red or white boiling potatoes
       ½ cup whole-wheat pastry flour
       ½ teaspoon paprika
        5 small boneless chicken breast halves, skinned
     1¼ cups defatted *chicken stock*
        1 large onion, chopped
       ¾ cup chopped mushrooms
       ½ cup chopped green pepper
       ½ cup chopped celery
        3 large cloves garlic, minced
    ½–1 tablespoon soy sauce
       ⅛ teaspoon cayenne pepper
       ½ cup dry white wine
        1 16-ounce can diced tomatoes in juice

Place the potatoes in a steamer basket in a pot of boiling water and cook, covered, for about 20–25 minutes or until potatoes are almost tender when pierced with a fork. Remove the potatoes from the pot, cool briefly, then peel and halve lengthwise. Combine the flour and paprika in a shallow bowl, mixing well. Coat the chicken breasts with the flour mixture, one at a time, by rolling them in the flour. Shake off excess flour and set the chicken aside.

Bring the chicken stock to a boil in a large skillet. Add the onion, mushrooms, green pepper, celery, and garlic. Cook the vegetables over moderate heat for 5 minutes, stirring occasionally, then add the soy sauce, cayenne, and chicken breasts. Reduce heat, cover, and simmer for 5–10 minutes, lifting cover to stir occasionally, if needed. Stir in the wine and tomatoes. Arrange the potatoes around the chicken, cover, and simmer for 25 minutes, or until the chicken and potatoes are tender. Stir occasionally, basting the chicken and potatoes with the sauce. (If desired, after stirring in the wine and tomatoes, the chicken, potatoes, and sauce may be transferred to a baking dish and set in a 325° oven to bake for 25 minutes until chicken and potatoes are tender.)

Makes 5 servings.

OVEN-BAKED BREADED CHICKEN

Either boneless chicken breasts or breasts with the bone in produce good results with this recipe.

Breading:
- ⅓ cup whole-wheat pastry flour
- ¼ cup canned evaporated skim milk
- 2 egg whites, beaten lightly
- ½–1 tablespoon soy sauce
- 1½ teaspoons lemon juice
- 1½ teaspoons onion powder
- ½ teaspoon garlic powder
  Dash cayenne pepper
- 1⅓ cups fine whole-wheat bread crumbs (from acceptable bread), plus 1½ teaspoons onion powder

- 4 small chicken breast halves, skinned

Combine all the breading ingredients except the bread crumbs and the onion powder in a bowl; stir well to mix. Prepare the bread crumbs by processing the bread in a processor or blender with the onion powder. Place the seasoned bread crumbs in a separate bowl. Coat each breast by dipping in the flour mixture, then in the bread crumbs, covering both sides. Arrange the chicken on a nonstick baking pan. Cover the pan with aluminum foil and bake in a 375° oven for 35 minutes. Remove foil, turn heat up to 425°, and continue baking another 15–20 minutes to crisp the coating.

Makes 4 servings.

ALTERNATIVE ENTRÉES

When you'd like a change to fish, pasta, or other dishes, look to these recipes.

OVEN-BAKED BREADED FILLET OF SOLE

We wanted to devise a recipe that was as close as possible to the fried fish fillets most people adore. This is the excellent result.

Breading:
- ⅓ cup whole-wheat pastry flour
- ¼ cup canned evaporated skim milk
- 2 egg whites, fork-beaten
- 1 teaspoon lemon juice
- 1 teaspoon onion powder
- ¼ teaspoon garlic powder
- 1⅓ cups fine whole-wheat bread crumbs (from acceptable bread) plus 1 teaspoon onion powder

About 8 fillets of sole, total weight about 1 pound

Combine all the breading ingredients except the bread crumbs and onion powder in a shallow bowl; stir to mix well. Prepare the bread crumbs by processing the bread in a processor or blender with the onion powder. Place the bread crumbs in another shallow bowl. Coat the fillets by dipping them, one by one, in the flour mixture and then in the bread crumbs, covering both sides. Arrange the fillets in a nonstick baking pan. Bake uncovered in a 350° oven for about 30–35 minutes (the breading should be browned and crisp-looking). Serve plain or with *Mustard-Yogurt Topping* (page 194).

Makes 4 servings.

CREOLE-STYLE FISH

Prepare the sauce and use it to make your choice of two different recipes: 1. Pour the sauce over serving-sized pieces of fish in a baking dish, then bake for about 30 minutes; or 2. dice the fish and drop it into a pot of simmering sauce to cook for about 15 minutes. Serve the diced fish and sauce over cooked brown rice, or with *Mashed Potatoes* (189).

You can use many different kinds of fish with this basic recipe. If you are going to dice and simmer the fish in the sauce, select a firm white fish such as halibut or bass. They also make excellent choices for baking. You can use red snapper, ling cod, haddock, or other fish for baking as well.

Creole Sauce:
- ½ cup vermouth
- 2 large onions, coarsely chopped
- 2 green peppers, coarsely chopped
- 1 cup diced celery with leaves
- ¼ cup chopped parsley
- 1 28-ounce can Italian plum tomatoes, undrained and coarsely chopped

1 cup canned tomato sauce
1 bay leaf
1 teaspoon curry powder
1 teaspoon spice blend such as Spice Islands Bouquet Garni or
    Fines Herbes
Dash cayenne pepper

Place vermouth in a large skillet or pot, bring to a boil, and add the onions, green peppers, celery, and parsley. Reduce heat, and sauté the vegetables for about 10 minutes, or until tender, stirring frequently. Add the tomatoes, tomato sauce, and all the seasonings, bring to a boil, then lower heat and simmer for about 25 minutes, stirring from time to time as required to prevent sticking.

Makes about 7 cups.

Recipe I: Baked Fish with Creole Sauce

1⅓ to 1½ pounds bass, halibut, or other fish of choice, cut into
            6 serving pieces
       3 cups *Creole Sauce* (there will be sauce left over)

Place the fish pieces in a baking dish, and pour about ½ cup of the sauce over each piece. Bake in a 375° oven, uncovered, for about 20–30 minutes, or until fish appears white and opaque when flaked lightly with a fork.

Makes 6 servings.

Recipe II: Fish Simmered in Creole Sauce

          1 recipe *Creole Sauce*
1⅓ to 1½ cups bass, halibut, or other firm white fish, diced

Bring the sauce to a boil in a large pot, reduce heat, and add the diced fish. Cover and let simmer for about 15 minutes.

Serve fish and sauce over cooked brown rice or *Mashed Potatoes* (page 189).

Makes 6 servings (8 cups).

LOBSTER SZECHUAN STYLE *
(or Scallops or Tuna Szechuan Style)

While lobster may be your preferred choice for making this dish, you can also get good results by substituting 1 cup cooked scallops, coarsely shredded, or 1 cup canned tuna, coarsely flaked.

½ cup chopped dried mushrooms, soaked in water for 10 minutes, then drained, *or* ½ cup chopped fresh mushrooms
⅓ cup chopped green onions (white part only)
2 cloves garlic, minced or crushed
1 teaspoon grated fresh ginger
1 cup cooked lobster chunks, coarsely shredded
¼ teaspoon hot dried crushed red pepper (*or*, for a less hot sauce, use a seeded dried red pepper, removing it at end of cooking period)
1⅓ cups defatted *chicken stock*
¼ cup dry sherry
1 teaspoon soy sauce
1 tablespoon cornstarch

Place a medium skillet over moderate heat and add the mushrooms, onions, garlic, and ginger; stir constantly for about 1 minute. Add the lobster and pepper. Stir in the stock, bring to a boil, lower the heat, and simmer for 2 minutes. Mix the sherry and soy sauce into the cornstarch to make a smooth paste. Add the cornstarch mixture to the skillet, stirring constantly until sauce is thickened. Serve with hot cooked brown rice.

Makes 2–3 servings.

SPAGHETTI WITH SAUCE

A hot dish of spaghetti topped with a tasty sauce makes a fine, filling meal. Three very different sauce recipes follow. The first is made by converting survival staple *Tomato-Veggie Stew* into an Italian-style sauce with a few simple additions. (You can also use the stew just as is for a satisfactory pasta topping.) The second, *Bolognese Sauce,* is an excellent meat-based tomato sauce, usually made with ground beef. You can get equally good results substituting ground turkey breast. The third, *Mushroom Cream Sauce,* is a delicious departure from the tomato-based sauces, and is also very good when served over baked, broiled, or poached fish, or over crêpes.

     2 cups cooked whole-wheat pasta (about 4–5 ounces uncooked)
     1½ cups Sauce I, II, or III (recipes follow)

Garnish: sprinkling of Sap Sago cheese (optional)

Makes 1 serving.

SAUCE I. SPAGHETTI SAUCE WITH TOMATO-VEGGIE STEW *

     1 28-ounce can Italian plum tomatoes, coarsely chopped
     1½ tablespoons dried Italian herb seasoning
     2 teaspoons garlic powder
     1½ teaspoons onion powder
     3 cups *Tomato-Veggie Stew*
     ¼ cup dry red wine
     1 tablespoon frozen apple juice concentrate (or more, if a sweeter sauce is preferred), optional

Place tomatoes and dry spices in a large pot. Bring to a boil and stir in the *Tomato-Veggie Stew*. Return to a boil, turn heat low, cover, and simmer for about 20 minutes, stirring occasionally as required. Add the wine about 5 minutes before the end of the cooking period. (If a smoother sauce is preferred, before adding the wine, place part of the sauce in a blender and purée it, then return blender contents to the pot; or you may purée the canned tomatoes or part of the *Tomato-Veggie Stew* in a blender at the start of the cooking.)

Makes about 6 cups.

SAUCE II. BOLOGNESE SAUCE

¾ pound ground raw turkey breast or very lean beef
1 teaspoon chile powder
1 teaspoon oregano
1 teaspoon rosemary
  Dash cayenne pepper
1 small onion, chopped
3 cloves garlic, minced or crushed
¾ cup finely chopped celery
½ cup shredded carrots
1 cup dry red wine
1 28-ounce can Italian tomatoes, coarsely chopped in blender
2 cups canned tomato sauce

Place a large skillet over moderate heat, add the ground turkey or lean beef, and sprinkle the spices over the meat. Stir-fry the meat and spices for about 10 minutes, mixing well, and using the back of the mixing spoon to break up clumps of turkey or beef as they cook. Add the onions, garlic, celery, and carrots and stir-fry another 5 minutes until the vegetables are partially cooked. Stir in the wine, cover, and cook over moderate heat for 10 minutes. Add the tomatoes and tomato sauce, stir, bring to a boil, then lower heat and simmer, covered, for about 1 hour.

Makes 6½ cups.

SAUCE III. MUSHROOM CREAM SAUCE*

3 cups defatted *chicken stock* or vegetable stock
1 cup sliced mushrooms
2 tablespoons canned tomato paste
2 teaspoons minced pimientos
1 teaspoon finely minced parsley
2 teaspoons soy sauce
2 teaspoons onion powder
4 tablespoons cornstarch
½ cup canned evaporated skim milk
¼ cup dry white wine

Put all the ingredients except the cornstarch, milk, and wine in a saucepan. Bring to a boil. Turn down the heat and simmer covered until the mushrooms are tender. In a separate bowl, mix the cornstarch, milk, and wine, blending well. Add the cornstarch mixture to the simmering sauce and stir constantly until thickened.

Makes about 4 cups.

PITA PIZZAS

Pita bread makes very satisfactory pizza crust. Using this recipe, you can quickly transform small-size pita breads into delicious individual pizzas, or cut the pizzas into dainty pie-shaped pieces for party appetizers. If you don't use all the pizzas, freeze the extra ones; or make only as many pizzas as you want, and freeze the leftover sauce for later use.

8 small whole-wheat pita breads

Pizza Sauce:
½ onion, quartered
3 cloves garlic, coarsely chopped

½ teaspoon Italian herb seasoning
½ teaspoon oregano
¼ teaspoon anise seed
1 15-ounce can tomato sauce
1 tablespoon cornstarch

Vegetable-Cheese Topping:
For *each* pizza, prepare the following:

¼ cup cottage cheese (1% or less fat, by weight)
3 thin slices onion, separated into rings
¼ cup chopped green pepper *and/or* 1 mushroom, thinly sliced
   Sprinkling of Sap Sago cheese
¼ teaspoon Italian herb seasoning

Prepare the sauce by placing all the sauce ingredients in a blender; blend until smooth. Transfer blender contents to a saucepan, heat to a boil, then reduce heat to low and simmer for about 10 minutes, stirring occasionally.

Separate each pita bread at the edges to make two rounds, stacking one round on top of the other, smooth sides down, and arrange the eight double-layer crusts on a baking sheet. (Doubling the crust adds flavor and body; but if you prefer, you can use only one round per pizza.) Spread on top of each of the eight crusts about ⅓ cup of the sauce, and then the cottage cheese. Distribute the vegetable toppings and end with the Sap Sago cheese and Italian seasoning. Bake in a 350° oven for 20 minutes, or until pizzas are just starting to brown.

Makes 8 individual pizzas.

VEGETABLE CURRY

½ cup white wine
1 large onion, sliced
2 cloves garlic, finely minced
1 cup vegetable stock or water
3 large tomatoes, quartered and blended in blender

1   potato, peeled and cut into chunks
3   turnips, peeled and quartered
2   parsnips, peeled and cut into chunks
1   rutabaga, peeled and cut into chunks
2   carrots, cut into chunks
1   stalk celery, chopped
2   apples, cut into chunks
¼   cup raisins
¼   cup chopped parsley
¼   cup canned pineapple juice
2   tablespoons curry powder
1   tablespoon soy sauce
3   tablespoons arrowroot (optional)

In a soup pot, pour in the wine and sauté the onions and garlic over medium heat, stirring occasionally, until they are tender. Add the tomatoes and stock and bring to a boil. Add the potato, turnips, parsnips, and rutabaga, cover, and cook over low heat until the potato is almost tender. Add the carrots, celery, apples, raisins, and the rest of the ingredients, except the arrowroot. Cover and simmer over low heat for about 20 minutes. If thickening is desired, make a paste of the arrowroot with ⅓ cup water, stir into the pot, and cook a little longer until thickened. Serve with hot cooked brown rice and *Cucumbers with Yogurt* (page 180).

Makes 6 servings.

CHEESE QUICHE

We think real men—and women, too—will like this delicious quiche.

1   cup fine whole-wheat bread crumbs (from acceptable bread —that is, whole-grain wheat bread without oil)
2   tablespoons canned tomato juice
1   carrot, very thinly sliced

1 green pepper, chopped
5 mushrooms, thinly sliced
1 large clove garlic
⅓–½ cup nonfat milk, as required
¼ cup frozen apple juice concentrate
3 cups cottage cheese (1% fat or less, by weight)
4 egg whites

Prepare the bread crumbs by processing bread in a food processor or blender. Mix the tomato juice with the bread crumbs and press the mixture into a 9-inch pie pan to form a crust approximately ¼-inch thick. Bake the crust at 350° for 10–15 minutes. Set the crust aside.

Place the carrots, green pepper, mushrooms, and garlic in a steamer basket and let them steam over boiling water in a covered pan for 10 minutes. Remove the garlic and place it in a blender with the milk and the apple juice. Add the cheese to the blender. (If using a moist-type cheese, place it in a strainer and rinse it first until the rinse water runs clear and only the dry curds remain. If using a dry-curd or pressed dry-curd cheese, such as hoop cheese, rinsing is not necessary.) Blend until smooth but still thick, adding more milk, a tablespoon at a time, if needed to achieve desired consistency. Transfer the cheese mixture to a bowl and add the steamed vegetables. Beat the egg whites until stiff peaks form and fold them into the cheese/vegetable mixture. Pour the quiche batter into the prepared crust and bake at 350° for 20–25 minutes. Let the quiche set for 15 minutes at room temperature before serving it.

Makes 6 servings.

Presliced turkey breast in small packages may be purchased at the poultry section of the supermarket for use in the two recipes that follow. It's a convenient way to prepare turkey, and delicious, too.

TURKEY BREAST SLICES IN WINE-CAPER SAUCE

If desired, steamed potato halves may be placed in the skillet with the turkey slices near the end of the cooking period, to finish cooking with the turkey slices. Spoon the sauce over the potatoes when putting them in the skillet.

    6 raw turkey breast slices (about 2½–3 ounces per slice)
    ¾ cup vermouth or other dry white wine
    ¾ cup bottled white grape juice
    ¾ cup water
    3 tablespoons lemon juice
    2 tablespoons Dijon-style mustard
    1 tablespoon arrowroot
    1 tablespoon coarsely chopped capers, drained
    ½ teaspoon onion powder
    ¼ teaspoon garlic powder

Pound the turkey slices with a mallet to tenderize them. Place them with ¼ cup water in a large skillet. Bring to a boil; then turn down the heat and simmer, covered, for 5 minutes. Turn the turkey slices over and add the wine, grape juice, and water. In a small bowl, combine the lemon juice and mustard, stirring well, and add 1 tablespoon water to dilute slightly. Blend in the arrowroot until smooth. Add this mixture to the skillet together with the remaining seasonings, stir, and return to a boil. Reduce the heat to low, cover, and cook for 35 minutes. During the cooking period, turn the slices over again once or twice, and stir gently to keep them covered with the sauce and to prevent sticking. Serve garnished with lemon slices and parsley sprigs.

Makes 5–6 servings.

Recipes 171

TURKEY-"FRIED" STEAK *

Mashed Potatoes (page 189) with *Onion Gravy* (page 190) would be a perfect accompaniment for this excellent sliced turkey recipe.

    1 cup fine whole-wheat bread crumbs (from acceptable bread)
    1 tablespoon onion powder
    1 teaspoon garlic powder
    ½ teaspoon paprika
    ⅛ teaspoon cayenne pepper
    6 raw turkey breast slices (about 2½–3 ounces per slice)
    ½ cup canned evaporated skim milk or nonfat milk (or water)
    ¾ cup water
    ½ cup dry white wine
    2 teaspoons soy sauce
    1 cup defatted *chicken stock* or vegetable stock (or water)

Prepare the bread crumbs by processing bread in a food processor or blender. Combine the bread crumbs with the dry spices and mix well. Pound the turkey slices with a mallet to tenderize them. Dip each slice in the milk, then in the bread crumbs, covering well. Reserve the leftover bread crumbs. Combine the water, wine, and soy sauce in a large skillet and bring to a boil. Lay the breaded turkey slices in the skillet and cook, covered, over medium heat for 8–10 minutes. Transfer the turkey slices to a baking dish and sprinkle them with the leftover bread crumbs. Place the stock in the skillet, bring to a boil, stir, and pour the skillet contents over the turkey slices. Cover and bake in a 400° oven for 20 minutes.

Makes 5–6 servings.

The two healthy burger recipes that follow deserve your consideration. The *"Little Beef Burgers"* are made with a small amount of beef stretched with buckwheat (kasha). The resulting burger is quite authentic in appearance, and makes a good burger substitute especially when eaten in a whole-wheat bun with the "fixings"—lettuce, tomato, sliced onion, and mustard or *Burger Sauce* (recipe follows). The *Turkey-Mushroom Burgers* are a low-calorie alternative burger for any runners still wanting to lose a few pounds.

"LITTLE BEEF BURGERS"

- ½ cup roasted buckwheat kernels, medium granulation (Wolff's Kasha)
- 6 ounces fat-trimmed flank steak, ground
- 1½ cups chopped onions, divided into two portions
- ⅔ cup chopped mushrooms
- 1 teaspoon soy sauce
- ¼ teaspoon garlic powder
- ¼ teaspoon cayenne pepper
- ⅓ cup potato flour (or, if preferred, rice or wheat flour)

Bring 1 cup water to a boil. Add the buckwheat, cover, and cook over low heat for 10 minutes. Turn off heat, keep covered, and let sit to permit kernels to swell. Place the flank steak in a skillet over medium heat and cook the meat, stirring constantly, until the pink color is gone. Add one portion of the onions and the mushrooms and continue to cook, stirring constantly, for another 4–5 minutes. Add the rest of the onions and the seasonings to the skillet and mix well, then combine with the buckwheat. Stir in the potato flour. Shape the mixture into 6 patties and lay them on a nonstick baking sheet. Broil until browned, about 15 minutes. Serve with *Burger Sauce*.

Makes 6 patties.

Burger Sauce:
- 1 cup canned tomato sauce
- ⅓ cup canned tomato paste
- ¼ cup water
- 1 tablespoon frozen apple juice concentrate

1 teaspoon cider vinegar
1 teaspoon soy sauce
1 teaspoon dry mustard
¼ teaspoon garlic powder

Place the ingredients in a blender; blend to mix well. Keep refrigerated.

Makes 1½ cups sauce.

TURKEY-MUSHROOM BURGERS

To make this recipe, you could purchase a small package of turkey breast slices and ask to have it ground.

2 cups ground raw turkey breast
2 cups chopped fresh mushrooms
1 cup chopped canned water chestnuts
¼ cup finely chopped onions
¼ cup finely chopped celery
1 canned chili pepper, finely chopped
2 teaspoons Dijon-style mustard
2 teaspoons poultry seasoning
3 egg whites

Combine all the ingredients except the egg whites. Beat the egg whites until stiff; fold into the other ingredients. Shape into patties and broil on a nonstick pan, turning once. Serve hot or cold with Dijon-style mustard, lettuce leaves, sliced tomatoes, and sliced onion.

Makes about 16 patties.

SOUPS, SALADS, AND VEGETABLES

A word of warning to runners about soups, salads, and vegetables, in general. Don't go overboard on them. As a runner, you need to eat plenty of higher-calorie complex-carbohydrate foods, keeping soups, salads, and most vegetables in a subordinate role. These foods tend to be low in calories, yet fill you up, with the result that you can easily drop below your optimal weight. Soups, even thick ones, do this because their watery base dilutes their calories; salads and vegetables tend to have the same effect because they give you lots of low-calorie bulk.

Don't have large portions of soup daily if you're happy with your present weight. Likewise, one large green salad with an abundance of raw vegetables per day is quite enough, unless you have pounds to lose. Enjoy the recipes for these foods that follow, but do be aware of their general tendency to cause weight loss if emphasized in the diet.

SPLIT PEA SOUP

Most recipes for split pea soup call for cooking the soup for an hour or longer. It's not necessary, and destroys some of the lovely color and fresh flavor of the peas. This delicious split pea soup cooks for only 25 minutes.

        8 cups water (or use vegetable stock if you have it)
    1⅓ cups split peas
    1½ cups chopped carrots
        1 cup peeled and chopped potatoes
        1 cup chopped onions
     ½ cup chopped green pepper
     ½ cup chopped celery
        2 cloves garlic, minced
        1 bay leaf
        1 teaspoon soy sauce

Place all the ingredients in a large soup pot. Bring to a boil, reduce heat to low, cover, and cook for 25 minutes. Remove and discard the bay leaf. Transfer all the soup, except about 2 cups, to a blender. Blend until smooth, and return to the soup pot to be mixed with the unblended soup. Serve hot.

Makes 9 cups.

VEGETABLE-BARLEY SOUP

Turnips and turnip greens give this vegetable soup an especially appealing fresh flavor, but if you wish, you can test the soup near the end of the cooking period and, if desired, add some extra seasonings in the form of a little thyme or marjoram, soy sauce, or a tablespoon or two of chopped parsley.

½ cup whole barley
2 cups diced carrots
2 cups diced turnips
1 cup chopped turnip greens (tops)
1 large onion, chopped
¾ cup chopped celery
1 cup fresh or frozen cut green beans
1 16-ounce can diced tomatoes in juice

Bring 3¼ cups water to a boil in a soup pot and stir in the barley. Reduce heat, cover, and cook for 45 minutes. Add 6 cups water and all the other ingredients except frozen green beans, if used, and the tomatoes. (If the green beans are fresh, add them now with the other vegetables.) Stir and bring the soup to a boil, then lower the heat and cook, covered, until the vegetables are tender, about 45 minutes. Add frozen green beans, if used, and the tomatoes about 20 minutes before the end of the cooking period.

Makes about 10 cups.

ITALIAN PEASANT SOUP

¼ cup white wine
1 cup finely chopped onions
1 cup finely diced celery
1 cup finely diced carrots
1½ cups diced peeled potatoes
1½ cups diced peeled parsnips
8 cups vegetable stock or water, or a combination of the two
½ teaspoon thyme
2 teaspoons crushed garlic
1 tablespoon soy sauce
2 cups chopped kale

In a large soup pot, pour in the wine and sauté the onions, celery, and carrots over medium heat, stirring occasionally, until the vegetables are tender, or about 25 minutes. Add the potatoes, parsnips, vegetable stock, thyme, garlic, and soy sauce, stir, bring the liquid to a simmer, and cook, covered, over low heat, until potatoes are not quite tender, or about 15 minutes. Add the greens and cook 10 to 15 minutes longer. If desired, float some cut-up diced oven-toasted whole-grain bread in each serving bowl, adding the bread just before serving.

Makes 8½ cups.

CREAMY CORN SOUP

5 cups frozen corn kernels, divided
1 potato, peeled and sliced into ½-inch rounds
1 small onion, coarsely chopped
1½ cups nonfat milk
1 13-ounce can evaporated skim milk
1 2-ounce jar sliced pimiento, chopped
1 teaspoon dillweed
Dash cayenne pepper

Place 2 cups of the corn and the potato in a pot with 1 cup water. Bring to a boil and cook, covered, over medium heat for about 10 minutes. Transfer the corn mixture to a blender and add the onion and nonfat milk; blend until smooth. Set a double boiler top over a pot of boiling water (you can use a stainless-steel bowl for the double boiler top). Add the blender contents and stir in the evaporated milk. Cook for about 5–10 minutes. Stir in the pimiento, seasonings, and remaining corn. Simmer for another 5 minutes, stirring occasionally.

Makes 7–8 cups.

MINESTRONE *

This extra-thick *minestrone* is almost stewlike in consistency. If you prefer it less thick, thin the finished soup by adding more liquid (tomato or V-8 juice, vegetable stock or defatted chicken stock or water), or add only 2/3 cup beans. Bean juice adds flavor, so don't drain the beans that go in at the end.

    2 carrots, chopped
    2 stalks celery, chopped
    1 onion, chopped
    1 green pepper, chopped
    ¼ cup parsley, chopped
    1 28-ounce can tomatoes, coarsely chopped
  2½ cups stock (defatted *chicken stock* or vegetable stock) or
       water, or a combination of stock and water
    1 tablespoon garlic powder
    1 tablespoon Italian herb seasoning
    1 large zucchini, finely chopped
    ⅔ cup uncooked whole-wheat macaroni, *or* 1 cup cooked
       wholewheat macaroni or *cooked brown rice*
    2 cups *cooked kidney beans,* undrained

Place all the ingredients except the zucchini, macaroni or rice, and beans in a soup pot. Bring to a boil, turn down heat, cover, and cook over medium heat for about 20 minutes. Add the zucchini and uncooked macaroni and cook another 10 minutes. Add beans. If using cooked macaroni or cooked rice, add with the beans. Heat through. Serve hot.

Makes about 2½ quarts.

SALADS

Create your own basic mixed green salads out of assorted raw vegetables, using lots of dark green lettuce. Choose a dressing from one of the group on pages 192–194, or use other suitable dressings.

Among the salad recipes that follow, we've included some main-dish salads, and also some made with grains—a way to eat salads and get your calories, too.

The salad that follows is basically a mixed green salad to which tuna and beans have been added to make it more substantial. You can use the recipe for making a basic mixed green salad by omitting the tuna, beans, and garnishes.

CHEF'S SALAD WITH TUNA AND BEANS *

Vary the vegetable ingredients in this salad to suit your fancy. Chopped watercress, bean or alfalfa sprouts, quartered tomatoes, sliced jicama, shredded carrots or red cabbage, or cooked vegetables such as cooked green beans would all be interesting additions.

Salad:
8 cups torn or chopped lettuce (romaine combined with another variety such as butter or red-leaf)

1 cup shredded iceberg lettuce (optional)
1 cup diced celery
½ cup sliced mushrooms
½ basket cherry tomatoes (halved, if large)
4 radishes, thinly sliced
½ small cucumber, sliced (peeled, if waxed)
½ small red onion, thinly sliced
½ cup canned tuna (water-packed), drained and flaked
½ cup *cooked garbanzo or kidney beans* (or a combination of the two), drained

Garnishes:
1 cup drained canned artichoke hearts (water-packed), quartered
1 cup sliced canned or home-cooked beets
1 red or green bell pepper, sliced in rings

Chill ingredients well. Combine salad ingredients in a large bowl, then add garnishes. Serve with *Creamy French Dressing* (page 193) or *Creamy Artichoke Dressing* (page 192).

Makes 4 servings.

CUCUMBERS WITH MOCK SOUR CREAM *

2 cups cucumber, peeled and thinly sliced
1 cup *Mock Sour Cream*
1 teaspoon dillweed
1 teaspoon caraway seed

Combine all ingredients in a bowl. Serve chilled.

Makes about 2½ cups.

CUCUMBERS WITH YOGURT

The combination of cucumbers, yogurt, and mint is particularly well-suited to accompany curry dishes, such as *Chicken Curry* (page 149) or *Vegetable Curry* (page 167).

    1 cup yogurt (1% or less fat, by weight)
    ½ cup finely cut green onions
    ¼ cup chopped fresh mint
    ¼ cup lemon juice
    2 cloves garlic, crushed
    2 cups cucumber, peeled and thinly sliced or diced

Combine the yogurt with all the ingredients except the cucumber, stirring to mix well. Add the cucumber (drain the cucumber first if watery) and toss thoroughly. If not served immediately, keep chilled in refrigerator and stir a few times to restore smooth consistency, if necessary, just before serving.

Makes about 2½ cups.

COLE SLAW *

Dressing:
    1 cup *Mock Sour Cream*
    ½ cup yogurt (1% or less fat, by weight)
    1 tablespoon onion powder

    6 cups grated cabbage (about ½ large cabbage)
    1 cup grated carrots
    1 8-ounce can crushed pineapple in own juices, drained (reserve ¼ cup juice)
    ⅓ cup raisins

Combine the dressing ingredients and set aside. Combine the cabbage and carrots in a large bowl. Stir in the drained pineapple and the ¼ cup reserved juice. Stir in the raisins and the dressing. Serve chilled.

Makes 6 cups.

POTATO SALAD

```
 5  russet or long-white potatoes
 2  hard-boiled eggs (discard yolks)
½  cup chopped celery
⅓  cup chopped green onions
 1  2-ounce jar sliced pimiento, chopped
1½  cups yogurt (1% or less fat, by weight)
1½  tablespoons Dijon-style mustard
 2  tablespoons onion powder
½  teaspoon dillweed
    Dash cayenne pepper
```

Place the potatoes in a vegetable steamer set over boiling water, cover, and steam until potatoes are just tender when pierced with a fork (or cook potatoes in boiling water until tender). Cool, peel, and place in refrigerator to chill while proceeding with the recipe. Chop one of the cooked egg whites, reserving the other for garnish. Combine chopped egg white, celery, green onions, and pimiento. In a separate bowl, combine the yogurt, mustard, onion powder, dillweed, and pepper. Stir the yogurt mixture into the vegetables. Slice the chilled potatoes and add them to the vegetables in the bowl, mixing gently. Transfer the salad to a lettuce-lined serving bowl and garnish with slices of the reserved egg white and a sprinkling of paprika.

Makes about 7 cups.

RICE SALAD *

If the cooked rice is hot when mixed with the dressing ingredients, it will absorb more of the flavors; so reheat it if it's cold (if you have time) before combining it with the dressing, then cool it a little before mixing in the vegetables.

Dressing:
   1 tablespoon dry mustard mixed with 1 teaspoon water
   ¼ cup vinegar
   1 tablespoon soy sauce
   Dash cayenne pepper

   2 cups *cooked brown rice* (see introductory note)
   2 green peppers, seeded and very coarsely chopped
   ½ cup sliced canned water chestnuts
   ¼ cup chopped red onion
   ¼ cup chopped parsley
   1 2-ounce jar sliced pimientos

Combine the dressing ingredients and mix with the rice. Stir in the other ingredients. Marinate in refrigerator at least 30 minutes. Serve chilled.

Makes 4 cups.

FRUITED RICE SALAD *

When summer fruits are available, it's an especially nice time to make this salad, although you can vary the fruits and make it any time of year. The salad is most attractive when freshly tossed, so don't combine rice and fruits in advance.

Marinade:
   2 tablespoons orange juice
   1½ tablespoons rice vinegar
   1½ teaspoons frozen orange juice concentrate
   ¼ teaspoon dry mustard

   2 cups cold *cooked brown rice*
   1 teaspoon chopped fresh mint
   2 nectarines
   2 plums
   1 peach
   1 small orange, sectioned and seeded
   1 cup green or red seedless grapes

Combine the rice and chopped mint in a large bowl; set aside. Slice the nectarines, plums, and peach (peel first, if desired), varying the shapes of the fruit slices for maximum eye appeal. Place the sliced fruit in another bowl. Add the orange sections, cut into halves, and the grapes. Stir together the marinade ingredients and combine with the fruit. Refrigerate for 15–20 minutes, stirring gently once or twice. Just before serving, toss the fruit and any marinade in the bowl with the rice. Serve in a lettuce-lined bowl garnished with strawberries and mint sprigs.

Makes 4 servings.

TABBOULI *

This grain-and-vegetable salad is almost a meal in itself. It uses bulgur wheat, a traditional grain of the Middle East. You can use the garnish of romaine lettuce leaves to scoop up the salad, Lebanese-style, if you wish.

   ½ cup uncooked bulgur wheat (finely milled preferred)
   1 cup defatted *chicken stock* or vegetable stock, or water, boiling hot

    2 tablespoons lemon juice
    ½ teaspoon soy sauce
    1 clove garlic, finely minced
      Dash cayenne pepper
    1 tomato, diced
    ½ cup chopped green onions
    ½ cup minced parsley
    ¼ cup finely chopped fresh mint
      Small romaine lettuce leaves (optional garnish)

Soak the bulgur in the hot liquid for 30 minutes. Combine the lemon juice, soy sauce, garlic, and cayenne in a small jar with a tight-fitting lid and shake vigorously to blend; set aside. Drain the bulgur and combine it with the tomato, green onions, parsley, and mint. Add the dressing and toss thoroughly. Serve chilled on individual salad plates with romaine lettuce garnish, if desired.

Makes 3–4 servings.

TROPICAL TUNA SALAD *

Dressing:
    ½ cup yogurt (1% or less fat, by weight)
    1 tablespoon prepared mustard
    1 teaspoon each: tarragon, curry powder, and onion powder
      Dash cayenne pepper

    1 7-ounce can water-packed tuna, drained and flaked
    1 20-ounce can crushed pineapple in own juices, drained
    1½ cups cold *cooked brown rice*
    1 cup chopped celery
    1 cup chopped green pepper
    1 large green onion, chopped

Combine the dressing ingredients in a small bowl. In a large bowl, combine the salad ingredients. Stir in the dressing, mixing lightly. Serve chilled.

Makes about 5 cups.

CHICKEN SALAD *

Expedite preparation of this recipe by using a food processor or even a blender, to finely cut the chicken and vegetables, but avoid chopping them too finely. Process the chicken, onion, and celery separately.

Dressing:
  ¾ cup *Mock Sour Cream* or yogurt (1% or less fat, by weight), *or,* preferably, *Mustard-Yogurt Topping* (page 194)
  1 teaspoon lemon juice (if not using *Mustard-Yogurt Topping)*

  2 cups rather finely chopped *simmered chicken*
  ¼ cup finely chopped onion
  ¼ cup finely chopped celery
  2 teaspoons chopped pimiento
  1 teaspoon caraway seeds

Combine the dressing with all the other ingredients, mixing well. Chill. (May be frozen.)

Makes 6 ¼-cup servings.

VEGETABLES

If you make your large daily green salad with various raw vegetables, including plenty of dark green lettuce, you may not even want to bother cooking vegetables outside of the

Tomato-Veggie Stew, your survival staple. That's okay, but we hope you'll make an exception and include potatoes and corn in your diet frequently. The two rank high among foods best-suited to the runner's diet, and are delicious and easily prepared.

There'll no doubt be times, however, when you'll want to prepare other cooked vegetables as well. An ideal way to cook any vegetable, both for nutrition and taste, is to steam it, because that method best preserves nutrients and flavor. To do this, you'll need a collapsible steamer basket that fits into a pot that can be covered. Set the basket into the pot that's partly filled with water, making certain the basket clears the top of the water. Bring the water to a boil, add the vegetables, and cover the pot. Cook for a few minutes or until the vegetables are tender-crisp, using the chart on page 187 as a time guide. Serve steamed vegetables plain, seasoned with herbs or spices, or topped with *Tomato-Veggie Stew*—good over cabbage, green beans, corn kernels, or summer squash such as zucchini—or with *Mustard-Yogurt Topping,* (page 194) which complements broccoli, asparagus, Brussels sprouts, or cauliflower.

Potatoes and corn are also delicious when steamed. Corn kernels or corn-on-the-cob steam in just 3 minutes. Red or white boiling potatoes, steamed whole in their jackets, take about 25 minutes. The other easy method of preparing potatoes is to bake them. Choose russets or Idaho baking potatoes, scrub them, prick with a fork in a few places to let steam escape, and set in a 400° oven for 40–45 minutes. They're done when they yield to a little pressure from your hand. To serve, peel steamed potatoes, or slit and press open baked potatoes, and top with *Mock Sour Cream* or yogurt (1% or less fat, by weight) and chopped chives or scallions. *Mustard-Yogurt Topping* and *Tomato-Veggie Stew* are also excellent over steamed or baked potatoes.

You'll find a few other ideas for potato preparations in the recipes in the next few pages.

FRESH VEGETABLE STEAMING TIMES

Fresh Vegetable	Minutes	Fresh Vegetable	Minutes
Asparagus	5	Kohlrabi, quartered	8–10
Beans (green, snap, or lima)	5	Leeks	5
Beets, quartered	15	Mushrooms	2
Broccoli	5	Okra	5
Brussels sprouts	5	Onions, whole	5
Cabbage, quartered	5	Pea pods (snow peas)	3
Carrots, ½-inch slices	5	Peppers, bell or chile	2–3
Cauliflower, florets	3	Potatoes, ½-inch slices	10
Cauliflower, whole	5	Potatoes, whole	20–25
Corn (on the cob, kernels)	3	Rutabagas	8
Eggplant	5	Squash, summer (zucchini, etc.)	3
Greens (kale, collards, spinach, etc.)	1–2	Tomatoes	3
		Turnips, quartered	8

OVEN-ROASTED POTATOES

Another simple method of preparing potatoes is to oven-roast them. In the three different versions of oven-roasted potatoes that follow, varying seasonings and styles of preparation give each a unique flavor. Use medium-sized red or white boiling potatoes in these recipes.

Version 1:
- 6 red or white boiling potatoes, peeled and sliced in half lengthwise
- 1 cup chopped onions
- 1½ tablespoons soy sauce

   1 teaspoon dried parsley
   1 teaspoon paprika

   Cut the potatoes into ¼-inch slices and line them up on a
nonstick baking pan. Sprinkle with the onions, soy sauce, and
the parsley and paprika. Bake covered at 400° for one hour.

Version 2:
   6 red or white boiling potatoes
   1 cup defatted *chicken stock* or vegetable stock
   1 tablespoon soy sauce
   1 tablespoon dry white wine
   1 tablespoon dried parsley
   ½ tablespoon paprika
   ¼ teaspoon onion powder
   ¼ teaspoon garlic powder
   Dash cayenne pepper

   Place potatoes in a steamer basket and steam, covered, over
boiling water for about 20–25 minutes or until potatoes are
almost tender when pierced with a fork. Cool potatoes, then
peel them and cut them in half lengthwise. Combine the stock
and other liquids and pour a little of the mixture on the bottom
of a nonstick baking pan. Arrange the potatoes on top, and
pour the remaining liquid over them. Mix the dry seasonings
and sprinkle them over the potatoes. Bake uncovered at 350°
for 20 minutes. (If the bottom of the dish becomes too dry,
add a little more stock or water.)

Version 3:
   6 red or white boiling potatoes
   ⅓ cup yogurt (1% or less fat, by weight)
   1 teaspoon onion powder
   1 teaspoon paprika
   Dash cayenne pepper

   Place potatoes in a steamer basket and steam, covered, over
boiling water for about 20–25 minutes or until potatoes are

almost tender when pierced with a fork. Cool potatoes, then peel them and cut them in half lengthwise. Arrange the potatoes in a nonstick baking pan. Combine the yogurt and spices with ¼ cup of water, and baste each potato with the mixture. Bake uncovered in a 400° oven for about 15–20 minutes, or until tops are golden.

Each version makes 6 servings.

MASHED POTATOES

4 large boiling potatoes
¾ cup canned evaporated skim milk (preferred), or nonfat milk, heated
2 teaspoons lemon juice
1 teaspoon soy sauce
1 tablespoon onion powder
1 teaspoon dillweed

Place the unpeeled potatoes in a large saucepan and cover them with water. Bring to a boil, lower the heat, and simmer, partially covered, until tender (about 35–45 minutes). Remove the potatoes from the pot, cool briefly, and peel. Mash them with a potato masher and whip in the milk and seasonings; then, using an electric or hand mixer, beat the potatoes until they are fluffy. Serve hot, plain or with *Onion Gravy* (recipe follows).

Makes 4 servings.

ONION GRAVY (for Potatoes) *

    1 teaspoon dried minced onions (or ready-toasted dried
        minced onions)
    1 cup defatted *chicken stock* or vegetable stock, or water
½–1 tablespoon soy sauce
    1 tablespoon cornstarch
    1 tablespoon whole-wheat pastry flour
  ¼ cup nonfat dry milk

To toast dried minced onions: place them in an aluminum-foil holder in a hot oven for a few minutes, stirring as needed, until lightly browned. Put the toasted onions in a saucepan with ½ cup of the stock and the soy sauce. In a small bowl, combine the cornstarch, flour, and dry milk, and blend in the other half-cup stock, stirring until smooth. Bring the contents in the saucepan to a boil; then stir in the cornstarch mixture. Reduce heat to low and cook, stirring constantly, until the gravy is thickened. If a thinner gravy is desired, stir in another ¼ cup of stock or water and simmer another minute.

Makes about 1 cup.

"FRENCH FRIES"

Recycle your leftover baked, boiled, steamed, or oven-roasted potatoes to make tasty mock fries using version 1; or start with uncooked potatoes and make them with version 2. Serve either version with bottled salsa or hot sauce.

Version 1:
  2 large cooked, peeled potatoes
     Onion powder (optional)
     Paprika (optional)

Slice potatoes and arrange the slices, separated, on a nonstick baking sheet. Bake in a 400° oven uncovered for 12–15 minutes. Turn the potatoes with a spatula and bake the other sides for another 5 minutes, or until golden brown. Sprinkle with onion powder and/or paprika, if desired, a few minutes before the end of the baking period.

Makes 1–2 servings.

Version 2:
   2 potatoes, peeled and cut into ½-inch wide slices
   1 tablespoon cornstarch
   1 tablespoon soy sauce

Soak the potato slices in 2 cups of water with the cornstarch and soy sauce for 10 minutes or longer. Drain. Arrange the potato slices on a nonstick baking sheet and bake in a 400° oven for 25–30 minutes, turning once to brown both sides.

Makes 2 servings.

STUFFED BAKED POTATOES *

Mock Sour Cream makes a wonderful topping for a baked potato, but you can also use it to make stuffed baked potatoes, as in this recipe.

Per Serving:
   1 baking potato
   ½ cup *Mock Sour Cream*
   1 tablespoon chopped green onion or chives
   ½ tablespoon grated Sap Sago cheese (optional)
   1 teaspoon onion powder
      Sprinkling of paprika or a spice blend, such as an Oriental or Mexican seasoning blend

Scrub potatoes, pierce each with a fork in several places, and place on a rack in a 400° oven to bake for 40–45 minutes, or until potatoes are done. (They should yield to pressure when squeezed lightly.) Slit the skin on one side along the length of each potato, leaving an inch at either end uncut; press to loosen contents, and scoop out the cooked potato from the shells into a bowl. Add the *Mock Sour Cream*, green onions or chives, Sap Sago cheese, if used, and onion powder, and mix well. Stuff each shell with the potato mixture and sprinkle a little paprika or spice blend over the slits in the shells. Place the stuffed potatoes on a baking sheet and return to a 375° oven to bake for 15 minutes or until heated through.

Makes 1 or more servings.

DRESSINGS, DIPS, AND SPREADS

Mock Sour Cream or yogurt provide the creamy base for *Creamy Artichoke* and *Thousand Island* dressings. The dressings tend to thicken a little after a few days in the refrigerator, but the desired consistency may be easily restored by whipping in a little nonfat milk or strained buttermilk.

CREAMY ARTICHOKE DRESSING *

1 cup *Mock Sour Cream* or yogurt (1% or less fat, by weight)
1 4-ounce can artichokes packed in water, well drained
1 clove garlic, coarsely chopped
½ teaspoon vinegar
½ teaspoon paprika
¼ teaspoon spice blend, such as Spice Islands Bouquet Garni
    Dash cayenne pepper

Place ingredients in a blender and blend thoroughly. Chill.

Makes 1½ cups.

THOUSAND ISLAND DRESSING *

1 cup *Mock Sour Cream* or yogurt (1% or less fat, by weight)
1 tablespoon canned tomato paste
2 tablespoons finely chopped green pepper
1 tablespoon finely chopped onion
¼ teaspoon garlic powder
  Dash cayenne pepper

Combine all ingredients and mix well. Chill.

Makes 1⅓ cups.

CREAMY FRENCH DRESSING

If you are wondering what to do with the extra baked yams in your refrigerator, try making this excellent French dressing!

1 cup peeled and mashed baked yams
¾ cup water
½ cup rice vinegar
3 tablespoons lemon juice
2 tablespoons canned tomato paste
1 tablespoon frozen apple juice concentrate
1 tablespoon soy sauce
½ teaspoon dry mustard
¼ teaspoon each: onion powder, garlic powder, and allspice
  Dash cayenne pepper

Combine all ingredients in a blender; blend until smooth. Chill.

Makes 2 cups.

VINAIGRETTE DRESSING

¼ cup apple cider vinegar
1 tablespoon lemon juice
1 cup water
2 teaspoons frozen apple juice concentrate
1 teaspoon soy sauce
½ teaspoon Dijon-style mustard
1 clove garlic, finely minced
1 tablespoon finely minced onion
1 teaspoon finely minced parsley
1 teaspoon finely minced chives
⅛ teaspoon paprika
Dash cayenne pepper

Combine all ingredients. Chill.

Makes about 1½ cups.

MUSTARD-YOGURT TOPPINGS

Dijon-style mustard and yogurt are the basic ingredients in two versions of a mustard-yogurt topping. The toppings may be used with baked potatoes, as a dressing over fish or cooked vegetables such as broccoli or cauliflower, or as a sandwich spread.

Version 1:
1 cup yogurt (1% or less fat, by weight)
2 teaspoons Dijon-style mustard
½ teaspoon garlic powder
¼ teaspoon dillweed

Combine all ingredients in a bowl. Mix well.

Makes about 1 cup.

Version 2:
 1 cup yogurt (1% or less fat, by weight)
 ½ tablespoon Dijon-style mustard
 ½ teaspoon each: rice vinegar, soy sauce, and garlic powder
 ½ teaspoon Angostura aromatic bitters (optional)
 ¼ cup finely chopped celery
 ¼ cup finely chopped red bell pepper

Combine all ingredients in a bowl. Mix well.

Makes about 1½ cups.

ONION DIP OR SPREAD *

Use this *Mock Sour Cream*-based recipe to prepare a spread for sandwiches or crackers, or serve it as a dip before a festive meal, along with celery and carrot sticks and other raw vegetables, and crackers.

  2½ tablespoons dried onion flakes
   1 cup *Mock Sour Cream*
 ½ to 2 tablespoons strained buttermilk, or yogurt (1% or less fat, by weight), according to thickness desired
   1 tablespoon lemon juice
   1 teaspoon onion powder
   ½ teaspoon garlic powder
   1 tablespoon dried parsley

Place the onion flakes on a piece of foil or small foil pan and set in a 375° oven for a few minutes to toast. Stir occasionally to brown lightly. Place most of the toasted onions in a blender, reserving about ½ tablespoon to add later. Add all the other ingredients, except the parsley and reserved toasted onion, and blend well. Stir in the parsley and reserved toasted onion. Chill.

Makes about 1 cup.

DEVILLED EGG DIP OR SPREAD *

Hard-boiled egg whites are blended with *Mock Sour Cream* and other ingredients in this "eggy"-tasting dip or spread. Vary the consistency to suit your purposes by modifying the amount of *Mock Sour Cream* you use; use more for a thinner consistency.

    4 cooked egg whites (discard yolks)
       About 1 cup *Mock Sour Cream*
    1 teaspoon curry powder
    1 teaspoon tarragon
    1 teaspoon grated Sap Sago cheese or soy sauce (optional)
    ½ teaspoon lemon juice
    ½ teaspoon Dijon-style mustard
       Dash Tabasco

Place all ingredients in a blender; blend until smooth. Chill.

Makes about 1 cup.

Use your cooked beans to make *Bean Spread* or *Hummus Dip*. Pinto or red beans are a good choice for the *Bean Spread*, and garbanzos are traditional in the Middle-Eastern *Hummus Dip*. Either makes a wonderful appetizer course accompanied with raw veggies, and with corn chips for the *Bean Spread*, and pita bread, cut into wedges, for the *Hummus Dip*. The *Bean Spread* also makes an excellent sandwich filling.

BEAN SPREAD *

    1 cup *cooked pinto beans, or other beans of choice,* drained
    ¼ cup yogurt (1% or less fat, by weight), or *Mock Sour Cream*
    ¼ cup chopped green onions
    1 tablespoon canned diced green chiles
    1 tablespoon onion powder

Dash cayenne pepper, or for a zingier spread, 1 teaspoon Mexican seasoning blend

Place the beans in a bowl and mash them. Stir in the other ingredients and mash again to combine well.

Makes about 1 cup.

HUMMUS DIP*

1½ cups *cooked garbanzo beans,* or 1 15-ounce can garbanzos, drained
 2 tablespoons lemon juice (fresh-squeezed preferred)
 1 clove garlic, coarsely chopped
 ½ cup minced fresh cilantro (Chinese or Mexican parsley), or 3 teaspoons dry cilantro

Purée all ingredients in a food processor or blender.

Makes 1¼ cups.

PIMIENTO CHEESE

Pimiento Cheese is an excellent sandwich filling and keeps well in the refrigerator. It may also be frozen.

 2 pepperoncini (bottled peppers in vinegar), seeds and stems removed
 1 2-ounce jar pimiento
 1 teaspoon onion powder
 ¼ teaspoon vinegar from pepperoncini jar
 ¼ teaspoon dry white wine
 1 cup cottage cheese (1% or less fat, by weight)

Finely chop one pepperoncini and set aside. Place the other pepperoncini and the remaining ingredients, except the cheese, in a blender and purée Add the cheese and blend until very smooth, stirring as required. Stir in the chopped pepperoncini. Chill.

Makes 1 cup.

SALMON PATÉ

Serve this elegant paté as an appetizer course along with raw vegetables and crackers, or use it as a delicious sandwich filling.

   1 7¾-ounce can pink salmon, drained
  ½ cup canned water-packed artichoke hearts, drained
   1 2-ounce jar pimiento
   1 tablespoon onion powder
   1 tablespoon garlic powder
1½ teaspoons chopped fresh dill, or 1 teaspoon dried dillweed
   1 teaspoon paprika
      Dash Tabasco
   2 cups cottage cheese (1% or less fat, by weight)

Remove skin and bones from salmon. Place salmon and the other ingredients, except the cheese, in a blender and blend well. Add the cheese, blending and stirring as required until the mixture is smooth and well blended. Chill.

Makes 2 cups.

BREAKFAST SELECTIONS, BREADS, AND MUFFINS

We suggest cooked whole-grain cereals for your standard breakfast fare. They're very filling and keep you going for hours. Two easy-to-prepare cereals are oatmeal and cracked wheat. Avoid instant oats which are overprocessed; the regular rolled oats cook fast enough.

COOKED ROLLED OATS

⅔ cup regular rolled oats
1½ cups boiling water

Stir the oats into briskly boiling water. Reduce heat to moderate and cook 5 minutes or longer, uncovered, until oatmeal has desired consistency, stirring near end as necessary. Cover, remove from heat, and let stand a few minutes. If you wish, add chopped, sliced, or grated apple or other fresh fruit, or a few raisins, to the cereal a few minutes before the end of the cooking period; cover and cook a little longer over low heat until fruit and cereal reach desired consistency. Serve plain or with toppings of hot or cold skim milk, sliced fresh fruit, and a sprinkling of cinnamon, as desired.

Makes 1 serving.

COOKED CRACKED WHEAT

½ cup cracked wheat
1½ cups boiling water

Stir the cracked wheat into briskly boiling water, reduce heat to low, cover, and cook for 7–10 minutes, stirring as necessary near the end of the cooking period; or cook in a double boiler over boiling water for 15–20 minutes. Serve with sliced fresh fruit or a few raisins, a sprinkling of cinnamon, and some hot or cold skim milk, if desired.

Makes 1 serving.

Store-bought granola is made with oil and seeds, but you can make your own Pritikin-OK *Granola* with the recipe below. Another dry cereal combination you can put together in seconds is *Apple-Oat Crunch,* which uses uncooked rolled oats as the base. They're popular in dry form in parts of Europe as a ready-to-eat breakfast food.

GRANOLA

⅓　cup raisins or currants
¾　cup water
4　cups regular rolled oats
¼　cup frozen apple juice concentrate
1　tablespoon vanilla extract
2　tablespoons whole-wheat pastry flour
2　tablespoons nonfat dry milk
1½　teaspoons cinnamon
⅛　teaspoon nutmeg

Soak the raisins or currants in the water for 20 minutes. Drain the raisins, reserving the water. Place the oats in a colander and pour the reserved water over them. Put the moistened oats in a mixing bowl and add the remaining ingredients, except the raisins or currants; mix well. Spread the granola in a thin layer on nonstick baking sheets. Bake in a

350° oven for 25 minutes. Add the raisins or currants to the granola for the last few minutes of baking.

Makes 5 cups.

APPLE-OAT CRUNCH

    1 cup regular rolled oats
    1 apple, sliced
    ½ cup unsweetened canned applesauce
    2 tablespoons raisins
       Dash cinnamon

Combine the uncooked oats and fruits, mixing well. Add the cinnamon.

Makes 1–2 servings.

Pritikin Pancakes are another excellent source of grains at breakfast. Use *Berry-Apple Compote* as a delicious pancake topping.

ORANGE-YOGURT PANCAKES

    1½ cups nonfat milk
     ½ cup yogurt (1% or less fat, by weight)
      2 egg whites
      2 cups whole-wheat pastry flour
     ½ cup fresh orange juice with pulp

Combine nonfat milk, nonfat yogurt, and egg whites in a blender. Add the flour and blend again. Add orange juice and blend briefly. Heat a nonstick skillet over moderate heat and pour the batter into the skillet to make pancakes of desired size. Bake until bubbles form on the top and the underside is browned; then flip over and bake until the other side is browned.

Makes 2–3 servings.

THREE-GRAIN PANCAKES *

If you wish, you can add 1 small diced banana and ½ cup frozen unsweetened blueberries (separated and drained of ice) to the pancake batter, after it has been blended.

    2 cups water
    1½ cups regular rolled oats
    1 cup whole-wheat pastry flour
    ¼ cup frozen apple juice concentrate, or 2 tablespoons raisins
    2 heaping tablespoons *cooked brown rice*
    1 scant tablespoon baking powder
    1½ teaspoons vanilla extract
    2 egg whites

Combine all the ingredients in a blender; blend until smooth. Heat a nonstick skillet over moderate heat, pour the batter on the skillet to make cakes of desired size, and bake until lightly browned on the underside. Turn and bake on the other side until sufficiently browned.

Makes 2–3 servings.

No death-dealing cholesterol-laden yolks in the egg recipes that follow. The yellow color in the first, *"Orange Eggs,"* comes from fresh orange juice; in the second, from a pinch of turmeric. These "scrambled eggs" will stick a little even when cooked in a nonstick skillet, so use a spatula or wooden spoon to ease them off the cooking surface. You could also, if you wish, wipe the surface of the skillet with a little oil, then wipe off the excess, to reduce sticking. Try either "scrambled egg" on top of a toasted whole-wheat English muffin, or surrounded by triangles of toasted whole-grain bread. Use the *"Fried Egg" Sandwich* for a quick brunch dish.

ORANGE EGGS

```
  4  egg whites
 ⅓  cup fresh orange juice with pulp
 ½  teaspoon soy sauce
  1  tablespoon nonfat dry milk
  1  teaspoon cornstarch
 ½  teaspoon onion powder
```

Combine egg whites, orange juice, and soy sauce in a bowl, whipping with a fork to mix well. Combine the dry ingredients and add to the egg mixture. Heat a nonstick skillet over moderate heat and pour in the mixture. Stir frequently to reduce sticking and cook for a few minutes to scrambled-egg consistency.

Makes 2 servings.

EGGS À LA LONGEVITY

```
  4  egg whites
1½  tablespoons nonfat milk
 ¼  teaspoon soy sauce
1½  tablespoons nonfat dry milk
 ¼  teaspoon cornstarch
 ⅛  teaspoon onion powder
     Pinch of turmeric
```

Blend egg whites, liquid nonfat milk, and soy sauce. Combine the dry ingredients and add to the egg white mixture. Heat a nonstick skillet over moderate heat and pour in the mixture. Stir frequently to reduce sticking, and cook for a few minutes to scrambled-egg consistency.

Makes 2 servings.

"FRIED EGG" SANDWICH

1 or 2 egg whites
    2 slices whole-grain bread of acceptable quality (made without oil)
      Lettuce leaves and tomato slices
      Dijon-style mustard and/or bottled salsa, optional

Heat a small nonstick skillet over low heat. Pour one or two egg whites over the bottom, letting them cover the surface. Let cook, without stirring, until the egg whites are almost set, then cover and let steam for a few minutes, turning off the heat. Spread a little mustard, if desired, over one of the slices of bread. Lift off the cooked egg whites with a nonstick spatula and lay over the mustard-spread bread. Spoon on salsa, if desired. Top with lettuce leaves, slices of tomato, and the other bread slice.

Makes 1 sandwich.

CORN BREAD

Rye flour, instead of the usual wheat flour, is used with the cornmeal in this corn bread recipe, for different flavor and texture.

1½ cups cornmeal (whole-grain, fine-grind preferred)
¾ cup rye flour (whole-grain preferred)
2 teaspoons onion powder
1 tablespoon baking powder
½ teaspoon baking soda
1½ cups strained buttermilk
½ cup water
2 egg whites, very lightly beaten

Combine dry ingredients in a bowl. Combine buttermilk and water and stir into the dry ingredients. Fold the egg whites into the batter. Pour the batter into a nonstick pan (9″ x 9″) and bake at 400° for 20 minutes, covered. If browning is desired, remove cover and place under the broiler for a couple of minutes. Remove from stove, cover until cool, then cut into serving squares.

Makes 12 servings.

OATMEAL BREAD

2 cups regular rolled oats
½ cup frozen apple juice concentrate
1 cup water
½ cup raisins, coarsely chopped
1½ cups whole-wheat or rice flour
1 teaspoon baking soda
1 tablespoon cinnamon

Combine the oats, apple juice, water, and raisins. Cover and allow to soak for 1 to 2 hours. Combine the flour, baking soda, and cinnamon and add to the mixture. Knead to a smooth, stiff dough. Shape into a round ½ inch thick and place in a 9-inch round cake pan. Using a knife, slash the top of the dough twice to mark off four equal wedges. Bake in a 400°

oven for 30 minutes; then reduce heat to 350° and continue baking for 10 minutes. Remove from oven, wrap in foil, and set on a wire rack to cool. Cut bread into quarters at slash marks; then cut each quarter in thin slices.

Makes one 9-inch round loaf (about 24 thin slices).

SWEET POTATO BREAD

Here's another use for leftover baked or boiled sweet potatoes or yams, when you get tired of putting them in your lunchbox.

1 cup mashed sweet potato or yam, cooled
¾ cup canned evaporated skim milk or nonfat milk
⅓ cup frozen apple juice concentrate
1 teaspoon soy sauce
1 tablespoon cinnamon
¼ teaspoon nutmeg
1 envelope active dry yeast, dissolved in ½ cup lukewarm water
4 cups whole-wheat pastry flour
1 tablespoon nonfat milk

Blend the potato, evaporated milk, apple juice, soy sauce, and spices in a food processor or blender. Transfer the mixture to a large bowl and stir in the dissolved yeast. Slowly add 3¼ cups of the flour, stirring to combine well. Knead for 3 to 5 minutes, gradually adding the rest of the flour. Shape into a loaf (the dough will be sticky), place in a nonstick loaf pan, and set the pan in a warm oven. (Preheat the oven to 150°, then turn off heat just before setting pan in it.) Let the dough rise for 1 hour. Bake in a 425° oven for 10 minutes; then prick the surface with a fork in several places and brush with the tablespoon of nonfat milk. Lower the heat to 375° and continue baking for 35 to 40 minutes. Cool before slicing. Cover bread with foil or plastic wrap to keep moist.

Makes 1 loaf (about 16 slices).

BANANA MUFFINS

Too many ripe bananas on hand? Make *Banana Muffins!*

        2 cups mashed very ripe bananas
      ½ cup canned evaporated skim milk
      ½ cup frozen apple juice concentrate
      ¼ cup strained buttermilk
    2½ cups whole-wheat pastry flour
        1 teaspoon baking soda
        1 tablespoon cinnamon
      ¼ teaspoon cardamom
        3 egg whites, beaten to form soft peaks

Combine the bananas and liquid ingredients. Combine the flour, baking soda, and spices. Mix the wet ingredients into the dry ingredients. Fold in the beaten egg whites. Pour the batter into nonstick muffin pans. Bake at 375° for 30–35 minutes or until done. Remove pans from oven and let sit for about 10 minutes before taking the muffins out of the pans.

Makes 16 muffins.

APPLE-OAT BRAN MUFFINS

        4 egg whites, lightly beaten
      ¾ cup nonfat milk
      ½ cup yogurt (1% or less fat, by weight)
      ¼ cup frozen apple juice concentrate
        1 cup regular rolled oats

  1 cup bran
  2 apples, peeled and grated
  ½ cup raisins or chopped pitted dates (optional)
  1½ cups whole-wheat pastry flour
  1½ teaspoons baking soda
  1 teaspoon cinnamon

Combine eggs, milk, yogurt, apple juice, oats, and bran, and stir to mix lightly. Stir in the apples and raisins or dates, if used. In a separate bowl, combine the flour, soda, and cinnamon, stirring to mix well. Add the dry ingredients to the fruit mixture, stirring lightly to combine well. Spoon into nonstick muffin pans and bake in a 425° oven for 25 minutes.

Makes about 24 muffins.

DESSERTS, BEVERAGES, AND SNACKS

BERRY-APPLE COMPOTE MERINGUE *

Berry-Apple Compote, a lovely dessert in itself, can be made into an elegant and airy baked meringue with the simple recipe below. You can also use *Berry-Apple Compote* to make a delicious "ice cream" (page 213). To make the meringue, let the compote cool a little before combining it with the beaten egg whites—it should be warm, *not hot.*

  1 recipe *Berry-Apple Compote,* any variety
  7 egg whites, beaten until stiff peaks form

Stir the warm (not hot) compote into the beaten egg whites and pour into a 9″ x 13″ glass or nonstick baking dish. Set the dish into a larger ovenproof pan filled with enough boiling water to reach about halfway up the sides of the baking dish.

Bake uncovered in a 375° oven for 25 minutes. Remove the baking dish from the water about 10 minutes before the end of the baking period, placing it directly on the oven rack to finish baking. The meringue should brown only slightly; if it begins to brown too much, let it finish baking with the oven door slightly open. Remove from oven and let set for about 10 minutes or longer before serving, or serve chilled.

Makes 10 servings.

DATE CAKE

      4 cups whole-wheat pastry flour
      1 tablespoon baking powder
      2 teaspoons baking soda
      4 teaspoons cinnamon
      2 teaspoons coriander
     ¼ teaspoon allspice
      6 egg whites
   1½ cups frozen apple juice concentrate
      1 cup canned evaporated skim milk
      1 tablespoon vanilla extract
     ½ 1-pound package pitted dates, chopped (about 1½ cups)

Combine the flour, baking powder, baking soda, cinnamon, coriander, and allspice in a large mixing bowl. Beat the egg whites until soft peaks form and stir into the dry ingredients. Combine the liquid ingredients and stir gently into the batter. Stir in the dates, making sure to break up clumps in order to distribute them evenly throughout the batter. Pour the batter into a 9″ x 9″ nonstick baking pan, and bake covered with an aluminum foil dome in a 350° oven for 35 minutes, removing cover for the last 15 minutes of baking. Remove the cake from the oven, cover, and cool.

Makes 10–12 servings.

CARROT-YAM CAKE

    4 cups whole-wheat pastry flour
    1 tablespoon baking powder
    2 teaspoons baking soda
    4 teaspoons cinnamon
    1 teaspoon allspice
    ½ teaspoon nutmeg
    6 egg whites
 1½ cups frozen apple juice concentrate
    ¾ cup canned evaporated skim milk
    1 tablespoon vanilla extract
    2 cups shredded carrots
    2 cups shredded yams

Combine the flour, baking powder, baking soda, cinnamon, allspice, and nutmeg in a large mixing bowl. Beat the egg whites until soft peaks form and stir into the dry ingredients. Combine the liquid ingredients and stir gently into the batter. Combine the carrots and yams and stir them into the batter, distributing evenly. Pour the batter into a 9″ x 13″ nonstick baking pan, and bake covered with an aluminum foil dome in a 350° oven for 40 minutes, removing cover for the last 15 minutes of baking. Remove the cake from the oven, cover, and cool.

Makes 16 servings.

PINEAPPLE-LEMON CHEESECAKE

Crust:
    1 cup fine whole-wheat bread crumbs (from acceptable bread)
    1 tablespoon frozen apple juice concentrate
    1 tablespoon water
    ½ teaspoon vanilla extract

Filling:
  2 8-ounce cans unsweetened crushed pineapple, juice-packed
  1½ packages unflavored gelatin
  1 cup frozen apple juice concentrate
  ¼ cup lemon juice
  2 cups cottage cheese (1% fat or less, by weight)
  ¾ cup strained buttermilk
  1 tablespoon vanilla extract
  1 egg white

Prepare the bread crumbs by processing bread in a food processor or blender. Mix the bread crumbs with the liquid ingredients for the crust and press the mixture into the bottom of a 10-inch pie pan to form a crust approximately ¼-inch thick. Bake the crust at 350° for 10–15 minutes. Let cool.

Drain the pineapple and combine the drained juices and the gelatin in a small bowl, mixing well. In a saucepan, heat the apple and lemon juices, add the gelatin mixture, and cook for 1 minute. Place the cheese in a blender. (If using a moist-type cheese, put it in a strainer and rinse it first until the rinse water runs clear and only the dry curds remain. If using a dry-curd or pressed dry-curd cheese, such as hoop cheese, rinsing is not necessary.) Add the buttermilk, drained pineapple, and vanilla, and blend thoroughly for 8–10 minutes until smooth. Add the blender mixture to the hot mixture. Beat the egg white until stiff peaks form and fold into the hot mixture. Pour the mixture into the crust and refrigerate to set.

Makes 8 servings.

Variation: PINEAPPLE-LEMON CHEESE-CAKE WITH BLUEBERRY TOPPING

Blueberry Topping:
  1 10-ounce package frozen blueberries (unsweetened)
  ¼ cup frozen apple juice concentrate

1 tablespoon cornstarch, mixed with 1 tablespoon water to make
  a paste
½ teaspoon vanilla extract

Prepare the pineapple-lemon cheesecake. Make the topping by placing the blueberries and apple juice in a saucepan. Heat to a boil over medium heat, and stir and mash the berries. Add the cornstarch mixture and continue stirring and heating until mixture is thickened. Stir in the vanilla. Let cool, then spread over the cheesecake after it has set.

BAKED APPLE CRUMB

4 apples, MacIntosh or Granny Smith, peeled and chopped
3 tablespoons raisins
1 tablespoon cinnamon
1 cup Grape-Nuts
¼ cup whole-wheat pastry flour
3 tablespoons frozen apple juice concentrate
¼ cup orange juice
1 grated lemon rind
3 tablespoons date sugar

Combine apples, raisins, and cinnamon in a bowl. Place in a 9-inch baking dish, covering the surface of the dish evenly. Combine the Grape-Nuts with the flour and apple juice and cover the apple layer. Mix the orange juice, lemon rind, and date sugar, and pour evenly over the crumbs. Bake in a 350° oven, covered, for 25 minutes; remove cover and continue baking for an additional 15 minutes.

Makes 6–8 servings.

RICE PUDDING *

```
  3 egg whites, fork-beaten
1⅓ cups canned evaporated skim milk
  ⅓ cup frozen apple juice concentrate
  1 tablespoon orange juice
  ⅓ cup currants
  1 teaspoon grated orange rind
  1 teaspoon vanilla extract
  1 teaspoon cinnamon
  ¼ teaspoon nutmeg
  2 cups cooked brown rice
```

Put all the ingredients except the rice into a bowl and stir to combine well. Mix in the rice. Transfer to a 1½ quart baking dish (a soufflé dish, if you have one) or a nonstick baking pan and bake in a 375° oven for 45 minutes, or until set and browned. Cool for 10 minutes or longer before serving, or serve chilled.

Makes 4–6 servings.

"ICE CREAM" *

To make this soft, delectable "ice cream," you'll need a food processor and frozen bananas. The bananas, sliced, go into the processor with a small amount of liquid or soft-solid liquid of your choice which flavors the bland but sweet bananas and helps to create the "ice cream" texture. Directions are provided for making several different varieties of "ice cream," but you could also invent your own, using various fruits or flavorings.

3 large *frozen bananas,* cut into large chunks

Additional ingredients for "ice cream" variety of choice, as follows:

"Ice Cream" Variety	*Additional Ingredients*
Vanilla	¼ cup yogurt (1% or less fat, by weight), and 2 teaspoons vanilla extract
Carob	½ cup strained buttermilk, and 1–2 tablespoons carob powder
Pineapple	1 8-ounce can crushed pineapple in own juices, undrained
Orange	1 large or 2 small sweet oranges, peeled and seeded with coarse membranes removed, cut into chunks
	½ teaspoon ground ginger
Berry-Apple Compote	½ cup *Berry-Apple Compote*
Pumpkin	1 cup canned pumpkin
	½ teaspoon pumpkin pie spice

Place the banana chunks in the processor with the additional ingredients to make the "ice cream" variety of your choice. Start blending, using a pulse action. (It may be necessary to remove the processor top and redistribute the bananas once or twice during the processing.) When almost smooth, process continuously for a few seconds more. Don't overprocess or "ice cream" will become too soft. Serve at once, or for a firmer consistency, freeze for 30 minutes to 4 hours in individual serving dishes covered with plastic wrap.

Makes 3 servings.

SMOOTHIES *

Make smoothies of any consistency—thick enough to require eating them with a spoon, if you like. The amount of liquid used in this recipe can be varied for the consistency you want and you can use whatever fruits and flavorings appeal to you. The one constant ingredient is a frozen banana, so keep plenty on hand to make this delectable treat.

> ½ cup, or more, liquid (unsweetened fruit juice; frozen unsweetened juice concentrate, diluted; nonfat milk; or strained buttermilk)
> 1 large *frozen banana,* cut into 1½-inch chunks
> ½ cup frozen unsweetened berries or other frozen unsweetened fruit
> ½–1 teaspoon vanilla extract (optional)

Pour liquid into a blender. Add the banana chunks and the rest of the fruit and the vanilla, if used. Blend until smooth, stirring as required. Add more liquid, if desired. Serve at once.

Makes about 1 cup (using ½ cup liquid).

FROZEN BANANA-ON-A-STICK

Here's another use for your ripe bananas. Coat them with the chocolatelike coating made with carob powder, then roll them in crushed cereal flakes to make a delicious frozen treat.

> ¼ cup carob powder
> ¼ cup frozen apple juice concentrate
> ¼ cup water
> 1 tablespoon nonfat dry milk
> 1 tablespoon vanilla extract
> 1 teaspoon arrowroot
> 2 large bananas, peeled
> 1 cup crushed cereal flakes (such as Nutri-Grain)

Place the carob powder, apple juice, water, dry milk, vanilla, and arrowroot in a saucepan over moderate heat. Stir constantly until the mixture thickens. Let cool. Cut the bananas in half crosswise and roll first in the carob paste, then in the cereal flakes, covering all sides. Insert a large toothpick at each end of all the banana halves, lay the bananas on a plate, and cover with plastic wrap. Place in the freezer, and let freeze hard before eating.

Makes 4 frozen bananas-on-a-stick.

GARBANZO NUTS *

Snack on these "beanuts" or add them to suitable recipes in place of nuts. If the cooked beans are frozen for a day or more before they're baked, they'll have an even better consistency when finished.

5 cups *cooked garbanzo beans*
    About 1 tablespoon each: onion powder and garlic powder

Place the beans in a single layer on a nonstick baking pan. While still damp, sprinkle the beans with the onion and garlic powder. Bake in a 350° oven for about 45 minutes, or until the beans are quite dry and browned. From time to time during the baking period, loosen the beans from the pan with a spatula and turn them by shaking the pan for more even browning.

Makes over 5 cups.

CORN CHIPS

By following the directions, you'll end up with 48 very symmetrical corn chips. But if neatness doesn't matter, just skip the knife-scoring step and lay the intact tortillas on the oven rack to crisp and lightly brown, then break into pieces.

6 corn tortillas

Using the point of a sharp knife, score each tortilla into 8 equal wedges as you would a pie. Start each cut an inch or more from the edge, pass through the center, and finish an inch or so from the opposite side. (The score marks will make it easy to break the tortillas, after baking, into neat wedge-shaped chips.) Place the scored tortillas on an oven rack or baking pan, avoiding overlapping, and bake in a hot oven until crisp and lightly browned, turning once or twice for even crisping. Break the crisped tortillas at the score marks into wedge shapes.

Makes 48 neat corn chips.

HOT CAROB

¼ cup cold water
½ cup nonfat dry milk
¼ cup carob powder
2 teaspoons dry Postum
2 cups boiling water

Place the cold water, dry milk, carob powder, and Postum in a blender. Blend until the dry ingredients look wet. Add the boiling water and blend at high speed for about 30 seconds, or until mixture becomes frothy and all the ingredients are well blended. Serve immediately.

Makes 2 servings.

HOT APPLE TODDY

Serve this marvelous and unusual beverage for breakfast or as a nightcap.

1 cup nonfat milk
1 cup unsweetened applesauce
½ teaspoon vanilla extract
¼ teaspoon cinnamon

Garnish: stick cinnamon (optional)

Put all the ingredients in a blender and blend at high speed until smooth and frothy. Heat mixture, but don't boil. Serve immediately in mugs garnished with cinnamon sticks.

Makes 2 servings.

PART THREE

WHAT THE RESEARCH SHOWS

10

Runners' Deaths

by Miles H. Robinson, M.D.

Much has been written about the tragic death of Jim Fixx, who died of a massive heart attack at the age of 52 while running alone last July on a country road in Vermont. My interest in this has been personal as well as scientific, having much enjoyed running the half-mile on varsity track teams in school and college. I understand what runners mean when they say it feels like flying; but it should not lead to dying.

Fixx was the author of two books on running,[1] the first of which has become a favorite reference for runners and one of the biggest sellers in publishing history. He wrote eloquently about the benefits which running and other exercise confer on mental and physical well-being. He practiced what he preached, running 80 miles a week for the last 15 years of his life. According to his family and friends, he developed a firm conviction that running would spare him the hard fate of his father, who had a heart attack at the age of 35 and died of another at 43. Fixx wrote in his last book:

Heart attacks, while not unknown in trained runners, are so rare as to be of negligible probability.[2]

The most extraordinary aspect of the stories about Fixx's death is how little attention the news media have paid to diet, the one thing which holds the greatest promise of preventing fatal heart attacks in runners and anyone else. In a long article in the *New York Times*[3] four days after his death, Lawrence K. Altman, M.D., learnedly discussed blockage of the coronary* arteries, medical and family history, smoking, blood pressure, stress tests, angiograms, and radioisotope outlining of the heart muscle. But not one word about diet appeared, and the article ended on the usual and, as we shall see, quite unnecessary note of mystery so common in medical articles for the lay public:

> Mr. Fixx's death is a reminder of how much more needs to be learned before heart disease can be conquered.

Let us consider first how much Jim Fixx knew about diet. From all accounts, he was a very intelligent man, an excellent writer of long experience, a former editor for the *Saturday Review, McCall's,* and *Life,* and his books give the impression of carefully covering all aspects of running. Early on, he seems to have had in mind the importance of making a change from the typical American diet, but this did not last:

> . . . his first wife, Mary Durling, claims that after he began running his diet changed from "a substantial breakfast to half an apple." Still, in a July 1979 interview in the *London Daily Mail,* Fixx described with some glee—and a certain arrogance—his breakfast that morning of fried eggs, sausage, bacon, buttered toast and coffee with cream. The meal was, of course, a horror of fats of the sort implicated in coronary heart disease. "If you run, you can

---

* Corona is the Greek word for crown. The network of arteries that nourish the heart muscle lie like a crown on the outside surface of the heart.

participate fully in the ways of our civilization and get away with it," he told the writer.[4]

The last sentence brings us to the very crux of the matter: his profound confidence in the ability of strenuous exercise to protect the heart. Where does this great faith come from, which betrayed Fixx and many others like him?

First, the public is surprisingly uninformed about what medical science has learned about heart disease, especially in the last ten years, from animal and clinical experiments and from epidemiological studies of population groups around the world. These studies have convinced almost all medical authorities that the most important cause of heart disease is the modern Western diet high in fat, with its accompanying excess of cholesterol which occurs only in animal food and cannot be burned up by exercise.

The study which had the most dramatic effect appeared 25 years ago, when a U.S. Army pathologist, Major William Enos, and his colleagues described autopsies on 300 American battle casualties in the Korean War.[5,6] In these young men averaging 22 years old, he found that there was coronary atherosclerosis * in 77% of the hearts, varying from fibrous thickening in 35% of the cases to large plaques completely blocking one or more major arteries in 3%. Enos pointed out that this was rare in Korean young men, and that 10,000 autopsies in Japan had shown that coronary disease was only one-tenth that in the U.S. He cited Davies'[7] finding that in Uganda grossly visible deposits in the coronaries are extremely uncommon and occur only in the well-fed African butcher.

The diet of the lower economic groups of both the Orient and Africa is close to the Pritikin diet, and thus quite different

---

* "Athero" and "sclero" are from the Greek words for gruel and hardness, respectively, and describe the mushy consistency of the fatty deposits which obstruct the artery, and the hardening and loss of elasticity of the artery itself.

from the high American consumption of meat and dairy products. In Japan, for example, the fat intake in 1919 was 5% of calories. As the country became more Westernized, this increased to 11% in 1960, 15% in 1965, and 17% in 1967.[8] It is now about 20%, still a far cry from our present 43%.

Enos concluded that one could state without reservation, but with some chagrin, that the coronaries of the young American male contain the best-fed fat-eating scavenger cells in the world. The significance of these cells, called foam cells, is that when regression of experimental atherosclerosis in animals is produced by taking the animals off a high-fat diet, the most consistent and dramatic change under the microscope is the virtual disappearance of these foam cells.[9]

The Enos report created a sensation in the medical-pathological world, and confirmation soon came from the U.S. Air Force. Flying personnel undergo an exacting physical examination for acceptance, and autopsies are required in all cases of death in military accidents. Rigal and colleagues[10] found that in these deaths, 70% of the airmen had some degree of coronary atherosclerosis and in 30% it was moderate or marked. The highest incidence in both categories was in men under 35 years of age.

It is generally acknowledged that the final cap on all this evidence was produced by the ten-year $150 million cholesterol study of the National Heart, Lung, Blood Institute,[11] reported in January 1984. It showed that for each 1% drop in blood levels of cholesterol, whether produced by diet or drugs, a 2% drop in the risk of a heart attack could be predicted.

In this connection, it should be noted that cholesterol is an indispensable ingredient of every cell, but our bodies automatically make all that we need. It is not true, as often alleged by those who are anxious to hang on to the excesses of our present rich meat-and-dairy diet, that eating cholesterol cuts down our own production of it. The scientific consensus now is that this feedback mechanism is absent or inconsequential in humans, and is characteristic only of animals like dogs, which have been designed by evolution to survive essentially on meat alone.

At the turn of the century, the amount of animal protein we ate was 52% of the total,[12] and it has since crept up to 68% in 1983.[13] The popular notion that we need to eat the large amount of animal protein we now consume is incorrect. If one eats enough whole grain to satisfy one's energy requirements, the average person will not be deprived of adequate protein.

The public unfamiliarity with new knowledge about diet and heart attacks, referred to above, is accentuated and perpetuated by a failing common to all of us, whether runners or not. Driven by a proper and admirable ambition to get the most out of life, we often tend to shut our eyes to relevant facts which would block a particular pleasure we like to enjoy—in this case, the indulgence in certain foods, the excess of which is bad for the arteries of most of us. The concept of a protective effect from exercise is, indeed, quite reasonable up to a point. However, we delude ourselves that exercise will completely protect us from the effects of a rich diet.

We still have a long way to go. The Western diet remains abnormally high in cholesterol and fat, derived from a high proportion of eggs,[14] dairy products, and saturated fat in meat from stall-fed livestock, all adding up to a fat intake of about 43% of total calories. We have a diet on which the arteries of only a small minority of individuals can remain healthy. Americans, characteristic of their adventurous spirit, have been doing better reforming their diets than many other Western countries. In the last decade, the U.S. death rate from heart disease has fallen about 25%, while in Britain it has actually increased slightly. Most authorities believe the chief cause of the U.S. improvement is the change in our diet. There has been a 10–15% reduction in consumption of foods high in total fat, saturated fat, and cholesterol, coincidental with a decline of 12–22% in the proportion of the population with high serum cholesterol levels.[15]

How can it be argued that our present diet is still abnormal for the human species? Few people seem aware of the strength of the case in favor of this position. Taking first a historical view, our current heavy emphasis on meat and dairy products is actually a radical change from the ancient human diet which prevailed since the dawn of civilization about 9,000 years ago, when grains in the form of unrefined bread were the "staff of life."[16] Porridge made from grain was the mainstay of both the ancient Greeks and Romans in their most productive era, when very few machines were used in industry and warfare, and superlative physical fitness was essential for survival. Cooked whole-grain cereal was the chief food of the Spartans, whose King Agesilaus campaigned hard in the field, not merely directing battles, at the age of 80; and of Sophocles, who wrote one of his great tragedies at the age of 90.[17]

Leonard Cottrell, the English historian, says that the Roman soldier rarely ate meat, and that according to Tacitus, the Roman historian, during the siege of Tigranocerta the soldiers only ate flesh-food when threatened by starvation.[18] In any case, only in the last two centuries has the Western world indulged in its present diet very high in fat, accompanied by an excess of cholesterol found only in food from animal sources. Eminent English authorities have pointed out that in 1770 the consumption of dietary fat was about 25 grams per day[19] and in 1880 it was 34 grams per day.[20] These figures amount to not over 11–15% of calories on a 2,000 calorie diet. This is one-third to one-quarter the fat which the average American eats. Even 70 years ago, the U.S. total intake of fat was about 32% of calories, three-quarters of what it is today.[21]

Fixx, in his last book, did not include diet among the "chief conditions that create heart attack risk."[22] His advice on fat was to limit it to 30% of calories. This at least takes us part way back, 70 years, on the historical scale of fat consumption, and is the recommendation of the American Heart Association, an organization considerably afflicted with an undue fondness for drug therapy, and rather lax about publicizing the full potential of diet in heart disease. The Pritikin diet goes all the way back, to the ancient diet of about 10% fat-calories.

Some doctors and lay people who yearn for a rich diet high in fat and cholesterol cite the famous Masai tribesmen who consume a good deal of milk and blood. So we must look at the interesting reasons why the Masai seldom have heart attacks. Over 50 autopsies by Dr. George Mann[23] of Vanderbilt Medical School have shown that the Masai have practically as much atherosclerotic plaque in their arteries as Western man, but the inside diameter of their coronary arteries is larger. Thus, the same size of plaque has less obstructive effect on the flow of blood to the heart muscle.

Mann attributed the larger diameter of their coronaries to the great amount of exercise taken by the Masai since childhood, particularly in the herding of cattle on foot, since it is well known that exercise increases the size of blood vessels. Mann put pedometers on the Masai and found that the young men walked an average of 18 miles a day, and the middle-aged men 12 miles. The old men walked six miles a day attending committee meetings.

Vermont's chief medical examiner, Eleanor N. McQuillen, M.D., found[24] the Fixx coronaries severely obstructed by atherosclerotic plaques of fat, cholesterol, and fibrous overgrowth. His left circumflex coronary artery was 97–99% blocked; the right coronary artery was 80–85% occluded; and the third coronary artery was 40–50% closed. His total blood cholesterol in 1980 was 253 mg/dl (people with under 160 mg/dl rarely have clogged coronaries), triglycerides desirably low at 57 mg/dl, and HDL cholesterol 87 mg/dl.[25]

How could Fixx and others like him run so well with clogged coronaries, until the last minute when the heart suddenly breaks down like the notorious "one-hoss shay"? As atherosclerosis slowly clogs the coronaries over months and years, the need of the heart for an adequate flow of blood in the capillaries lying alongside each single muscle fiber (an intimate blood supply for muscle found only in the heart), stimulates the growth of a *collateral* circulation of tiny arteries and capillaries which fan out ahead of the blockages in the main coronary arteries.

The collaterals are wonderful evidence of the tenacity with which our loyal hearts hang on to life, but these detours around the obstructions cannot accomplish as much as the original intact coronaries. There is a limit to the development of collaterals, and eventually the collective obstruction of the main coronary arteries becomes so widespread that the sources for the collaterals do not provide enough blood to nourish the working muscles of the heart. When that point is reached, usually precipitated by some extra stress, the result is an infarction,* or an electrical imbalance between the normal and abnormal portions of the heart bringing on a fatal arrythmia.

From what scientific source have Jim Fixx and other runners got the idea that running can provide immunity from heart attacks? The most prominent advocate of this theory in the medical profession has been Dr. T. J. Bassler, a pathologist and long-distance runner, who 12 years ago asserted that a search of the literature "had failed to document a single death due to coronary atherosclerosis among marathon finishers." [26] In 1978 he was reported declaring that "when the level of vigorous exercise is raised high enough, the protection from coronary heart disease appears to be absolute." [27] As recently as 1982 Bassler was quoted as saying that running would protect against a heart attack for five years in those who could run a sub-4-hour marathon and refrained from smoking; and that if deposits were already present in the arteries, running a total of 16,000 kilometers would remove the plaques and restore a free flow of blood in the arteries. [28] A great many jog-

---

* The word "infarct" is from the Latin, meaning to stuff into. The heart tissue, damaged by an inadequate supply of blood from clogged arteries, appears under the microscope to be stuffed with dead and dying cellular debris.

gers and other athletes have depended on these optimistic statements.

However, in 1980, in a scientific journal Bassler acknowledged that "No serious researcher should ever say that marathon running provides complete immunity from coronary-heart disease." He took the position that his theory depended on meticulous autopsies still to come:

> The "Bassler hypothesis" states that the marathon runner's lifestyle will protect against the aging process. Your ability to cover 42 km on foot is the best index of your life-style. No death in a marathon runner should be overlooked. Meticulous autopsies, such as those reported by Noakes et al., provide the only way to evaluate this hypothesis. [29]

Thus, there seems to be a marked discrepancy between what Bassler has said for popular consumption and what he has admitted in a scientific publication. As a runner himself, he naturally has a great emotional temptation to believe that running, which obviously has many physical and psychological benefits, can also prevent the insidious clogging of arteries caused by a diet unduly rich in fat and cholesterol.

Bassler's defense of his theory strains belief, as shown in the following exchange:

> Asked whether Fixx's death disproved his theory, Dr. Bassler answered only that eventually he would examine the medical reports. How long would that take? "Two years," suggested Dr. Bassler. "Maybe ten." [30]

Two or ten years to do what? The acute need of runners and other members of the public is not more research in this field, but a full and frank dissemination of what medical science *already* knows. This knowledge boils down to the conclusion that the basic cause of clogged coronary arteries is the modern Western diet.

Before we go further into the disconcerting evidence of what a rich diet does to the heart, we should cheerfully keep in mind the extraordinary power of the body to repair damage, *provided* it is consistently presented with more favorable conditions. For example, Dr. L. E. Lamb,[31] formerly professor of medicine at Baylor and Chief of Clinical Sciences at the USAF School of Aerospace Medicine, has emphasized the work of Wissler on monkeys, Brant and colleagues on humans, and three decades of worldwide epidemiological studies, all of which suggest that "major diet changes can result in *reversal* of coronary artery disease."

In the opinion of Dr. William Castelli, director of the National Institutes of Health's famous Framingham Studies, "Diet could reverse coronary disease in 90% of the patients if we got everyone's cholesterol below 150 mg/dl."[32] Dr. Antonio Gotto, president of the American Heart Association, has expressed essentially the same opinion: "If we lower the cholesterol count of everyone in the United States below 150, we could probably wipe out heart disease."[33]

Dr. Castelli had particularly strong reasons for his assertion. He went to medical school in Belgium after World War II, and was surprised to learn that two years of severe wartime restriction of fat, cholesterol, and calories in the diet had made it impossible for medical schools in Belgium, Holland, Norway, and Poland to find gross coronary lesions in autopsied hearts to show their students. The plaques had disappeared. The reason? The Germans had taken most of the livestock to Germany, and these occupied countries had to live largely on grain and vegetables. Prof. Gotthard Schettler of the University of Heidelberg recently reported in detail[34] the same phenomenon in Germany during that war, and he also ascribed it to the severe scarcity of fat and its accompanying cholesterol. After the war, as the rich diet returned, he observed a great resurgence in coronary deaths.

These facts show vividly how much promise there is in changing one's diet. The extraordinary results that can be achieved take time, partly because the cholesterol pool in the body is only slowly depleted. The turnover time for cholesterol in human atherosclerotic tissues ranges up to 2½ years.[35] Six months to a year are the shortest times for atherosclerotic regression that have been reported.[36]

Let us now look further at more of the sobering evidence which may inspire us to eat a better diet. Before Jim Fixx died, there were numerous poignant reports in the lay press of fatal heart attacks while jogging. Jim Shettler, 42, a runner for 25 years and winner of the National AAU Masters 25-kilometer run, died while on a short run, the day after running 23 hilly miles.[37] Jim Dooley, 37, the city official who oversaw the expansion of Anaheim Stadium for the Los Angeles Rams, died while jogging near his home.[38] Robert Clarke, 49, a physiologist, died when he stopped to rest before continuing up a hill on his regular 3–4 mile daily run.[39] Col. Giles Hall, 50, USAF Director of Health Professions Recruiting for the Air Force in Randolph, Texas, a daily jogger for 20 years, died while jogging.[40]

Dr. Robert Summers, longtime administrator of the Miami Heart Institute, dropped dead while jogging.[41] Dr. Edward Lauth, 46, a proponent of the jogging program which he helped a local Heart Association to institute, died while jogging around Miami Beach's La Gorce Country Club.[42] Dr. David Doroff, 49, a clinical psychologist active throughout his life, joined the jogging boom in 1978, completed an 18-mile training run for the New York City Marathon, had a negative exercise test by his cardiologist, and dropped dead of a heart attack in the cardiologist's office. Autopsy revealed two of the coronary arteries 90% occluded, and the third 60% blocked.[43]

One of the most prominent marathoners was Congressman Goodloe Byron, who died suddenly while on a 15-mile training run in 1978. According to his wife, he knew his heart was impaired, but believed in Bassler's theory, and "saw running as his way to stay alive." [44]

Heredity, and other features of life-style, such as smoking, play a role in atherosclerosis, but in the vast majority of cases none has the overall importance of diet. Vuori et al. examined the circumstances surrounding 2,606 sudden deaths,[45,46] and found that 73% of them were caused by acute or chronic coronary artery disease. At least one-third were associated with physical or psychological stress. Sudden deaths in connection with sporting activities or regular daily routine were rare, but there was a considerable risk of sudden death associated with strenuous physical exercise in subjects with manifest or *latent* cardiac disease, especially if there had been no gradual increase in exercise and training.

Pain in the front or back of the chest which develops during running is a serious sign which should be investigated. Noakes and Opie, from the Ischemic Heart Disease Laboratories of the University of Cape Town and Groote Schuur Hospital in South Africa, describe the case of a 35-year-old runner with these symptoms who died suddenly two hours after a short period of surfing during which he felt breathless.[47,48] He had had a three-week period of exertional chest pain with ST-depression (abnormal reading on electrocardiograph) on a treadmill test. Opie also described two other men who dropped dead, one a 19-year-old who died during a marathon. The other died suddenly after a 6–8-mile run, having previously undertaken several 20-mile runs. At autopsy, both of these had coronary obstruction, markedly so in the second case.

Opie's review of 21 sudden deaths in athletes found that 18 died of heart attacks either during or after sport, and that there was firm or strongly suggestive evidence of coronary heart disease in 16 and suggestive clinical evidence in 2. As a group, these subjects tended to be smokers; to have a family history of early heart attacks; and to have had antecedent symptoms of chest pain or pressure, fatigue, or blackout. Psychological factors were thought to be important in 8, since hormones of the adrenalin family may precipitate spasm of coronary branches in the heart muscle and arrythmias.[49] From his review of the literature (35 references), Opie concluded that the risk of sudden death is very serious if there is chest pain, pressure, or undue tiredness before, during, or after sport.

Jim Fixx had these symptoms. His second wife, Alice, recalled one day in 1980, after he had been working in the yard:

> Jim had the classic symptoms of heart trouble. He had to stop, lie down, he couldn't move. He was sweating, short of breath, nauseated, pain in the chest. After it passed, he just went about his work. . . . He really was negligent in that area and rarely went to a doctor.[50]

Lamb has emphasized that most American men over 40 years of age have a *silent* disease of coronary artery obstruction, which may not prevent marathon running or even show up in electrocardiograph-treadmill testing:

> Then one day a little fatty-cholesterol deposit bursts like a pimple or tears and a clot may form in the artery. After that occurs if you exercise, then you may indeed work your heart muscle beyond its blood supply and a fatal heart attack may occur. . . . Most of the young U.S. Army men who died while exercising had clots in a coronary artery that had been there for a day or longer before the exercise even occurred. . . . As many as one-third of all heart attacks are silent.[51]

Lamb pointed out that exercise may not cause a heart attack, and exercise may not prevent a heart attack. "Safe exercise" will help prevent heart disease, but unwise use of exercise could be dangerous, and the way to improve the safety of exercise is to relieve or reverse the disease in the coronary arteries. He recommended that until the blood cholesterol and blood pressure in a middle-aged man have remained at optimal low levels for three months, together with a ban on smoking, the only unsupervised exercise that should be permitted is walking and light calisthenics, and this should *never* be done at a pace so fast that it prevents carrying on a conversation at the same time.

Waller and Roberts at the National Heart, Lung, and Blood Institute, studied clinical and autopsy data on five white male runners aged 40 to 53 years, two of whom had been marathon runners. None had clinical evidence of cardiac disease before becoming a habitual runner, and all of them died while running. At autopsy, all had severe (greater than 75%) atherosclerotic luminal narrowing of their major coronary arteries. Of the five, at least four had hypercholesterolemia, which was greater than 300 mg/dl in three of the men; 240 mg/dl in one; and no figure available for the fifth man.[52] These high blood cholesterols indicate the high-fat, high-cholesterol diet of these men.

Two subjects had hypertension, one had angina pectoris, and none had clinical evidence of an acute myocardial infarct. Only one had symptoms, which consisted of episodes of pain beneath the sternum with radiation to the left arm after he had run about 13 kilometers. This pain would disappear after walking about 100 feet, and then he could run another 19–26 kilometers without further pain. He was the only one with a positive stress test, consisting of electrocardiographic ST-depression without pain. He had no angina when he started running at age 39, but it appeared 8 years later, 2 years before death.

Four of the five runners had healed (clinically silent) myocardial infarcts. The authors concluded that "coronary heart disease appears to be the major killer of conditioned runners aged 40 years and over who die while running."

W. Kannel, former director of the NIH Framingham study,[53] believes that "the key to the prevention of sudden deaths remains the reduction of risk of coronary attacks," especially since 60% of these deaths occur in persons who have manifested no prior indications of coronary disease known to either the patients' families or their physicians.

What are the statistical risks of a heart attack for joggers as compared with nonjoggers? P. D. Thompson et al. studied 12 men who died during jogging in the state of Rhode Island from 1975 to 1980. In 11 of these the cause of death was coronary heart disease (CHD), while one died of an acute gastrointestinal hemorrhage.[54] The prevalence of jogging among men aged 30 through 64 in Rhode Island was determined by a random-digit telephone survey. The incidence of death during jogging was one death per year for every 7,620 joggers, or approximately one death per 396,000 man-hours of jogging. It is of great importance that this rate is seven times the estimated death rate from CHD during more sedentary activities in Rhode Island.

As one looks over reports of runners' deaths, it is surprising how rarely they contain anything about the diet of the runner. Except for Lamb's reference to animal, clinical, and worldwide epidemiological work, suggesting that major dietary changes can reverse coronary disease, none of the foregoing reports about runners, whether made by medical professionals or by laymen, have shown any real interest in what the runners were accustomed to eat. The extensive research findings of diet-induced atherosclerosis have not really penetrated the consciousness of most of the physicians who are interested in the sudden deaths which take place in sports. That being the case, we can hardly blame Jim Fixx, other runners, or the news media for their neglect of this vital subject.

An unfortunate practice which sidetracks and lulls people into complacency about their diet are the outdated standards for blood levels of cholesterol which are still found on most medical laboratory report sheets. Few, if any, set a maximum safe value of less than 240 mg/dl, and usually considerably higher. For example, the Smith Kline Laboratories in January 1984 gave a top normal figure of 240 mg/dl for persons under

30 years of age, and 330 mg/dl for those over 50. The twelve branches of the Reference Laboratory in Southern California in October 1984 listed the normal range as 150–330 mg/dl without respect to age. These are not valid normal values, but simply averages currently found in the whole American population which is substantially afflicted with atherosclerotic disease. This situation is well known to the highest research authorities in our National Heart, Lung, Blood Institute:

Thus, 20 years ago there were sufficient data [from other countries] to cast serious doubt on the validity of standards commonly accepted in the United States for normal serum* cholesterol concentration. They indicated that a lifelong pattern of diet was inducing chronic hypercholesterolemia in a majority of Americans, contributing decisively to widespread atherogenesis. They further suggested that optimal serum cholesterol levels, for optimal freedom from atherosclerotic disease over an optimal life span, were considerably lower than those common in the United States population, due to the nature of the diet. Such optimal levels prevailed among only a minority of Americans fortunate enough to have the endogenous metabolic regulatory mechanisms that enabled them to maintain low serum cholesterol levels while habitually ingesting a diet high in cholesterol and saturated fats.[55]

The persistence of misleading "normal" laboratory values epitomizes the conservative reluctance of many sectors of the medical profession to accept the full significance and inevitability of the dietary revolution which is now taking place.

The false assurance conveyed by these values is well shown by the results of the Chicago Heart Association nine-year study of 12,000 men reported last year.[56] It found the following relation between total blood cholesterol and number of deaths due to heart disease per 1,000 persons:

* Cholesterol tests are done on the serum of the blood, which is the liquid part left after removal of the red blood cells.

CHOLESTEROL LEVEL mg/dl	*Relative Risk of*	
	Developing Heart Disease	*Dying of Heart Disease*
	FRAMINGHAM STUDY*	CHICAGO HEART ASSOC.†
140–159	(114–193) 1	1
160–179		4.5
195–218	5.3	6.3
219–240	6.7	7.5
241–268	12.4	8.5
268+	15.3	16.5

* *Lancet*, Aug. 1982 † *Medical World News*, April 1983

These figures, together with many other studies, lead to the conclusion that the best goal for a safe blood cholesterol level is 100 plus one's age.

As mentioned earlier, except for a minority of persons who have an unusual hereditary ability to manage excess fat and cholesterol, the hearts of most Americans are far more susceptible to heart attacks than they need to be, simply because evolution did not design the arteries of humans to cope with the modern Western diet.

In the last ten years, careful scientific research has confirmed what many pioneers in the field of health and full of common sense have known for centuries, long before the modern processing of food and the unlimited availability of dietary fat existed.[57]

Our ideas about food for humanity have come full circle. The perfect diet is out there. All we need is the will to reach out for it. Like many good things in this world, it is a mixture of wholeness, simplicity, and restraint.

Notes for Chapter 10

1. Fixx, James F., *The Complete Book of Running*, Random House, 1977 (980,000 copies not including 16 foreign editions); *Jim Fixx's Second Book of Running*, Random House, 1980.
2. *Jim Fixx's Second Book of Running*, pp. 24, 196.
3. Altman, L. K., *New York Times*, July 24, 1984.
4. Pietschmann, R. J., *Runner's World*, November 1984, p. 42.
5. Enos, W. F. et al., *JAMA* 152:1090–1093 (1953).
6. Enos, et al., *Am. J. Cardiol.* 9:343–354 (1962).
7. Davies, J. M. P., *Lab. Investig.* 10:205 (1961).
8. *Diabetes Outlook*, 18:8, no. 1, (1983), citing Y. Goto, Professor of Medicine at Tohoku University School of Medicine.
9. St. Clair, R. W., *Medical Times*, 108:49–58 (1980).
10. Rigal, R. D. et al, *Am. J. Cardiol.* 6:19–25 (1960).
11. National Heart, Lung, Blood Institute, *JAMA* 251:351–374 (1984).
12. Friend, B. & R. Marston, *National Food Situation*, U.S. Dept. of Agriculture, Pub. No. NFSD-154 (1975), p. 28.
13. U.S. Dept. of Agriculture, unpublished data.
14. Molecular biology has recently shown that the cholesterol receptors on the cells of the average person cannot handle more than a total of 100 mg per day, the content of half a medium-size egg.
15. U.S. Dept. of Health & Human Services, *Prevention '82*, DHHS (PHS) Pub. No. 82-50157 (1982).
16. Leviticus 26:26.
17. Kitto, H. D. F., *The Greeks*, Penguin, 1957, pp. 33, 93.
18. Cottrell, L., *The Great Invasion*, Coward-McCann, New York, 1962, p. 73.
19. Burkitt, D. P. & Trowell, H. C., *Refined Carbohydrate Foods and Disease*, Academic Press, New York, 1975, p. 53.
20. Drummond, J. C., Wilbraham, A., & Hollingsworth, D. F., *The Englishman's Food*, Jonathan Cape, London, 1957, pp. 458–9.
21. U.S. Department of Agriculture, cited in *Nutrition Week*, April 26, 1984, p. 6.
22. *Jim Fixx's Second Book of Running*, pp. 24, 141.
23. Mann, G. V. et al., *Lancet* 2:1308 (1965).
24. Pietschmann, R. J., *Runner's World*, November 1984, p. 39.
25. Higdon, H., *The Runner*, November 1984, p. 35.
26. Bassler, T. J., *Lancet* 2:711–712 (1972).
27. Restak, R. M., *New York Post* (magazine section), October 29, 1978.
28. Sumner, J., *The Age*, Sydney, Australia, October 16, 1982.
29. Bassler, T. J., *N. Eng. J. Med.* 302:57–58 (1980).
30. Higdon, H., op. cit., p. 36.
31. Lamb, L. E., *The Health Letter* 13:1–4 (1979).
32. *Medical World News*, September 3, 1979.

33. Quoted in *New West,* February 4, 1977.
34. Schettler, G., *Preventive Medicine,* 12:75–83 (1983). On a lecture tour here 20 years ago, he told the same story, but perhaps few understood its full significance (see *Medical Tribune,* December 15, 1969, p. 21).
35. Editorial, *Lancet* 2:614 (1976).
36. Knight, L. et al. *Surg. Forum,* 23:141–2 (1972); Starzl, T. E. et al., *Lancet,* 2:940–44 (1973); Henderson, R. R., & Rowe, G. G., *Am. Heart J.* 86:165–72 (1973); Barndt, R., Jr. et al., *Ann. Int. Med.* 86:139–46 (1977).
37. Henderson, J., *Runner's World,* September 1976.
38. Dodson, M., *Los Angeles Times,* June 12, 1981.
39. Lamb, L. E., op. cit.
40. *Aviation, Space, and Environmental Medicine,* June 1979, p. 656.
41. Bloom, M., *Medical World News,* November 27, 1978.
42. Editorial, *Medical Tribune,* 19:18 (1978).
43. Bloom, M., op. cit.
44. *Joggers* X:1,5 (1978).
45. Vuori, I., et al. *Cardiology* 63:287–304 (1978).
46. Danilevicius, Z., *JAMA* 240:1754–1755 (1978).
47. Noakes, T. D. & Opie, L. H., *Medical World News,* June 27, 1977, p. 53.
48. Opie, L. H., *N. Eng. J. Med.* October 30, 1975, pp. 941–942.
49. Opie, L. H., *Lancet* 1:263–266 (1975).
50. Higdon, H., op. cit., p. 35.
51. Lamb, L. E., op. cit.
52. Waller, B. F. & Roberts, W. C., *Am. J. Cardiol.* 45:423 (1980).
53. Check, W. A., *JAMA* 246:581–589 (1981).
54. Thompson, P. D. et al. *JAMA* 247:2535–2538 (1982).
55. *Report of the Working Group on Arteriosclerosis of the National Heart, Lung, Blood Institute.* Pub. No. NIH 82-2035 (1981), p. 274.
56. *Medical World News,* April 11, 1983, p. 15.
57. Henry, M. (1662–1714). "It was a common saying among the Puritans, 'Brown bread and the Gospel are good fare.' " in *Bartlett's Quotations,* Little Brown & Co., 1937, p. 188.

11

The Scientific Basis
for the Diet

Degenerative diseases, such as diabetes, heart disease, hypertension, and breast and colon cancer, are still widely assumed to be a natural aspect of getting older as the body "degenerates." If this is true, we are confronted with explaining why these diseases are essentially limited to the most developed and, theoretically, the most scientifically advanced populations in the world. In my view, these conditions are not diseases, but symptoms of chronic metabolic injury resulting from the highly processed, artificial diet eaten in developed areas, principally from excessive amounts of cholesterol and fat in our diets.*

A toxin is any substance that when taken in excess can cause death. Cyanide is very lethal, but the minute amount found naturally in lima beans rarely causes adverse effects. We can assume that the amount of cyanide in lima beans is far

* Chapter 11 is modified from a guest editorial in Preventive Medicine 11, 1982. Copyright © 1982 by Academic Press, Inc. All rights of reproduction in any form reserved. Reprinted by permission.

below the toxic level. In contrast to cyanide, iron is necessary to maintain life; but even so, excess iron intake can cause iron overload of the liver and result in death. In Africa, the Bantu use iron pots and get three to five times as much iron as the amount specified in the U.S. Recommended Dietary Allowances (RDA). In these days of megavitamins, this may not seem much, but the excess reaches a toxic level creating iron overload of the liver in 75 percent of the males and 25 percent of the females, resulting in unnecessary deaths.

In the amounts in which they are consumed in Western countries, cholesterol and fat reach toxic levels. It is this toxicity that I hold responsible for the degenerative diseases—pathological processes resulting from aberrations in the intake and metabolic processing of cholesterol and other lipids.

In 1955, when my cholesterol level hovered around 300 mg/dl, fueled by my daily ingestion of 700 mg of cholesterol, physicians assured me that it was in the high normal range, that my diet was excellent, and that stress and heredity were my principal heart-disease risk factors. Nevertheless, I soon developed coronary insufficiency so advanced that I was advised to completely limit all exercise. In retrospect, this circumstance may have been fortunate, saving me from a possible infarct resulting from the vigorous tennis matches in which I engaged at the time.

For 20 years prior to this I had been following closely the epidemiology of cardiovascular and other degenerative diseases in the medical literature, although I had not applied this information to my own life-style. I had found that atherosclerosis is essentially nonexistent in populations with adult cholesterol levels below 150 mg/dl. A feature common to all these populations seemed to be a cholesterol intake of less than 100 mg a day.

During the late 1940s and early 1950s, Keys reported the findings of more than 25 investigations; without exception, he found heart disease to be rare in these low-cholesterol-consuming populations.[1] Of particular interest were Keys's analyses of populations—especially the Japanese—who lost their immunity to heart disease when they migrated to areas in which cholesterol and fat intake were higher, and adopted the new diet.

The Japanese are heavy smokers, yet this well-established heart-disease risk factor seems to be of significantly less importance in the presence of a low-cholesterol and low-fat diet. Although they are number one among the developed nations in salt intake, hypertension, and strokes, the Japanese incidence of heart disease is the lowest among the developed nations. A diet containing only 10 percent fat kept the average cholesterol level of this population at 150 mg/dl for years. Unfortunately, due to Western influence, fat intake has doubled and serum cholesterol and the incidence of heart disease have substantially risen.

In the United States, where the mean population cholesterol level exceeds 200 mg/dl, both smoking and hypertension substantially contribute to the development of heart disease. Perhaps the low Japanese cholesterol levels protect against the development of atherosclerosis in spite of these risk factors.

Among the populations that seem immune to heart disease is one close to our southern borders. Fifty thousand Tarahumara Indians, living in the isolation of the Sierra Madre Occidental mountains in northern Mexico, are part of a natural dietary experiment that has been going on for the past 2,000 years. Their athletic stamina—they can run up to 200 miles— has attracted the attention of a number of scientists. One of them, Dr. William E. Connor, has conducted a number of investigations of their diet and general health. He found no evidence of deaths from cardiovascular disease and concluded that their diet is typical of other populations among which heart disease is virtually nonexistent. Of their total caloric intake, fat makes up 10 percent (P/S = 2.0); protein, 13 percent; and carbohydrates, 75–80 percent. The diet provides 15– 20 g/day of crude fiber, only 75 mg/day of cholesterol, and meets all nutritional requirements. Adult cholesterol levels among the Tarahumaras range from 100 to 140 mg/dl.[2,3]

In 1955, when I decided to change my high-cholesterol, high-fat dietary lifestyle, I adopted a diet nutritionally identical to the Tarahumara and similar diets, though I prepared my food in a manner pleasing to my Western-trained tastes. This is the same diet I have been recommending for 25 years, although for those with cholesterol levels of 250 mg/dl or greater, I found it was more effective to limit cholesterol intake to 15 mg a day, until serum levels dropped below 140 mg/dl.

In less than three years on this type of diet, my cholesterol dropped to 100 mg/dl, and it has remained in that range for 25 years. In the last six years, my dietary recommendations have been incorporated into the nutritional service at the Longevity Centers, and on an average cholesterol levels of people there drop 27 percent in three to four weeks.

Serum cholesterol levels of people who come to the Longevity Centers—mostly white Americans—drop quickly on a diet nutritionally similar to the Tarahumara diet; conversely, when Tarahumara are given American intakes of cholesterol, serum cholesterol rapidly rises toward American levels.[4] The response seems universal.

Framingham data early indicated that "normal" cholesterol levels in the United States were normal only for a country where heart disease is rampant. Even the early Cleveland Clinic angiographic data destroyed the "normal" cholesterol-level concept.[5] Among 723 men 17 to 39 years old, significant (greater than 50%) coronary lesions were found to be directly related to cholesterol level even within the "acceptable" limits of serum cholesterol.

SIGNIFICANT CORONARY LESIONS ASSOCIATED WITH SERUM CHOLESTEROL LEVELS

SERUM CHOLESTEROL (mg/dl)	SIGNIFICANT LESIONS (> 50%) PERCENTAGE OF TOTAL CASES
<200	20
201–225	38
226–250	48
251–275	60
276–300	77

This growing mass of epidemiological evidence—all pointing in the same direction—was further illuminated by the findings of Brown and Goldstein, who were able to show the mechanisms involved in setting the safe limits of circulating serum cholesterol. To quote Michael Brown: "Why, therefore, is Western man oversaturating his receptors and depositing LDL cholesterol in his arteries?" To lower plasma levels of LDL (to ideal levels) requires a diet of less than 100 mg of cholesterol daily and thus excludes all meat products and eggs, "a diet which I would never eat, which allows almost nothing except nuts and berries."[6] I phoned Dr. Brown and said, "I have bad news for you: Nuts are not on my diet—too high in fat. All that's left is berries." It did not take long to explain that the marvelous recipes adapted from American and foreign cuisines would give him a wide-ranging fare free of the risks of high cholesterol and high fat intake. The question that arises is *Why is there such a reluctance to change the atherogenic diet?*

Henry Blackburn wrote a splendid article, "The Public Health View of Diet and Mass Hyperlipidemia,"[7] whose thesis can be summarized in three sentences: "Atherosclerotic CHD (coronary heart disease) is a public health phenomenon of affluent cultures. Population comparisons suggest that mass hyperlipidemia is a prime requisite for mass atherosclerosis. On the basis of available evidence, the habitual diet of a cul-

ture is, in turn, the chief factor leading to hyperlipidemia."
Blackburn divides the world into four categories according to
cholesterol levels, as shown below.

RELATIONSHIP OF MEAN POPULATION CHOLESTEROL LEVEL AND INCIDENCE OF ATHEROSCLEROSIS

MEAN POPULATION CHOLESTEROL LEVEL (mg/dl)	INCIDENCE OF ATHEROSCLEROSIS
120	Rare
160	Minimal
190	Reduced
220–280	Epidemic

He selects a mean population cholesterol level of 160 mg/dl as
the best compromise (minimal CHD, and good palatability),
and states: "Population total cholesterol averages above 200
mg/dl are found incompatible with optimal cardiovascular
health for populations." Other expert groups have concurred
with this general position. The American Health Foundation
Conference on "Health Effects of Blood Lipids: Optimal Distributions for Populations" made an optimal recommendation
of 160 mg/dl.[8]

But what Blackburn recommends to the U.S. public with its
average serum cholesterol of 220 mg/dl is the American Heart
Association (AHA) diet: 30 percent fat and 300 mg cholesterol
—because, he points out, large-scale studies have shown it is
able to produce cholesterol drops of 6–7 percent. A quick
calculation indicates that a seven percent drop from 220 mg/dl
still leaves those hapless individuals with excessively high levels of 205 mg/dl, which Blackburn himself stated is incompatible with optimal cardiovascular health. To achieve the ideal,
a mean population cholesterol level of 160 mg/dl, requires a

drop of 27 percent. On my recommended diet, this 27 percent cholesterol reduction occurs in a month.[9]

The hopelessness of the position of those who cannot see beyond the AHA diet is apparent also in a statement made by AHA spokesman Scott Grundy that the AHA diet could only reduce the mean cholesterol level of U.S. men to 200 mg/dl. He goes on to say: "Yet despite such a change, half the male population would have cholesterol concentrations over 200 mg/dl. Many workers believe that levels over 200 mg/dl are still too high for adequate prevention of atherosclerotic disease. Thus, it is doubtful that atherosclerotic disease in our society can be obliterated by diet control alone, and additional measures will have to be taken to rid the American population of this disease. The methods are currently not available and will have to be developed through new research.[10]

The conclusion that diet alone cannot reduce the mean serum cholesterol level below 200 mg/dl is true with the AHA diet, of course. But Grundy asserts that this 30-percent-fat, 300-mg-cholesterol diet is the most effective diet for lowering cholesterol level—which is not true. Since the AHA diet does not work, he blames this on "genetics" and says new methods not currently available will have to be developed through new research.

While health professionals knowledgeable about the dietary basis of CHD are unable to face up to the magnitude of the dietary changes that must be made to achieve adequate lowering of serum cholesterol, they are willing to use hypocholesteremic drugs that have been discredited because of the possible excess cancer risk they introduce; to subject hyperlipidemic patients to an ileal bypass that will reduce the cholesterol level little more effectively than a diet with less than 10 percent fat and 100 mg of cholesterol; and to continue to make dietary recommendations of 300 mg cholesterol and 30 percent fat when during 20 years of trials this diet has failed to reduce cholesterol levels adequately.

Worse yet, it should be noted that these dietary recommendations when first made to the nation in 1961 had not been adequately tested. Pearce and Dayton, who directed the eight-year Wadsworth Veterans Administration AHA diet trial with 846 men, commented, "It is important to remember that no population under study has been consuming a diet high in polyunsaturated fats over long periods of time." [11] After the Wadsworth study, Dayton said not only that he would not recommend a high-polyunsaturated (PUFA) diet to most of his patients, but that a diet of ten percent fat would be his choice. In the official report, the investigator wrote: "The diet tested in this program was selected for purely pragmatic reasons: we did not believe we could mount and sustain a trial of any other type of lipid-lowering diet in this institution. Epidemiological studies favor the conclusion that a low-fat diet is perhaps the promising path to longevity." [12]

Though high-PUFA diets fail to reduce the risk of heart disease, they may *enhance* the risk of cancer. The 1982 National Academy of Sciences report *Diet, Nutrition, and Cancer* concluded that a relationship between fat and cancer was most persuasive. [13] T. C. Campbell, one of the authors of the report, stated that if a diet is high in PUFA, total fat should be less than 20 percent of total calories because of the possible increased cancer risk. So convinced is Campbell of the danger of excess fat that he stated: "The relationship between diet and cancer, in my opinion, is now more persuasively established than the one between diet and heart disease."

What, then, was the recommendation that followed from this observation? Campbell continued: "We decided to come up with a reasonable, practical number, something the whole population might work toward. So we recommended a reduction in fat intake from a current 40% of total calories to 30%, although I would suggest getting it down to about 20%. In China, where I was in June, it's only 9%. So you can go down to 20% and not experience problems."

But the public recommendation is 30 percent! Cancer and heart-disease researchers are alike in their tendency to treat the public as though they were incapable of accepting an optimal dietary recommendation.

My experience with 15,000 people who have been through my centers and millions who have read or heard about my diet belies this underestimation of a large part of the public. Why shouldn't everyone who wishes to follow an optimal diet be informed on the facts and be encouraged to make the necessary lifestyle changes?

When people achieve rapid health improvement, as very many do on an optimal diet, they become motivated to continue permanently so as to maximize health gains and avoid regressing. My diet, combined with exercise, has been effective not only with patients with cardiovascular symptoms but with non-insulin-dependent diabetics, 75 percent of whom are off insulin in four weeks, including some who had been taking it for 20 years.[14] In four weeks, 85 percent of hypertensives on drug therapy are off medication, with normal blood pressure, on this same diet/exercise regimen. In three weeks, cholesterol and triglycerides drop 25–30 percent on the regimen. Compliance, considering the difficulties in pursuing this kind of dietary life-style in a milieu in which not even health authorities encourage it, is surprisingly good; over a five-year period, compliance varies between 50 and 75 percent.[15]

If health care authorities recommended that cholesterol intake not exceed 100 mg/day and fat intake not exceed ten percent of total calories, the benefits experienced by those who follow my program could be experienced by millions more. The benefits would extend not only to sick people; healthy, active people would also gain. Many world-class athletes are on my diet and are experiencing thrilling, new, higher levels of performance.

The experts, already in agreement on the biochemical goals, are now beginning to agree on the guidelines: Cholesterol intake needs to be under 100 mg/day and fat intake not over ten percent. Leading investigators—Seymour Dayton in coronary heart disease, T. C. Campbell in cancer, and J. W. Anderson in diabetes—are all looking respectfully at a ten-percent-fat diet, or are already using it.

New health recommendations from authoritative sources are also moving slowly in the direction of advocating optimal fat and cholesterol intakes. These are encouraging trends; but there are still many problems to be overcome in terms of facilitating widespread enactment of these dietary goals. Only by replacing "compromise" by "ideal" can we ever hope to achieve the optimal diet for maximum quality and duration of life.

Notes for Chapter 11

1. Keys, A., Kimura, N., Kusukawa, A., Bronte-Stewart, B., *et al.* Lessons from serum cholesterol studies in Japan, Hawaii, and Los Angeles. *Ann. Int. Med.,* 1958, *48*: 83–94.

2. Cerqueira, M. T., Fry, M. M., and Connor, W. E. The food and nutrient intakes of the Tarahumara Indians of Mexico. *Amer. J. Clin. Nutr.,* (1979), *32*:905–15.

3. Connor, W. E., Cerqueira, M. T., Connor, R. W., Wallace, R. B., *et al.* The plasma lipids, lipo-proteins, and diet of the Tarahumara Indians of Mexico. *Amer. J. Clin. Nutr.,* 1978, *31*:1131–42.

4. McMurry, M. P., Connor, W. E., and Cerqueira, M. T. Dietary cholesterol and the plasma lipids and lipoproteins in the Tarahumara Indians: A people habituated to a low cholesterol diet after weaning. *Amer. J. Clin. Nutr.,* 1982, *35*:741–44.

5. Page, I. H., Berettoni, J. N., Butkas, A., and Stones, F. M. Prediction of coronary heart disease based on clinical suspicion, age, total cholesterol and triglyceride. *Circulation,* 1970, *62*:625–45.

6. Carpenter, M. "Healthy" receptors can't handle even "normal" lipid. *Med. Tribune,* 1980, *21*:3, 19.

7. Blackburn, H. The public health view of diet and mass hyperlipidemia. *Cardiovasc. Rev. Rep.,* Aug. 1980, 433–42:Sept. 1980, 361–69.

8. Wissler, R. W., Armstrong, M., Bilheimer, D., *et al.* Conference on the health effects of blood lipids: Optimal distributions for populations. *Prev. Med.,* 1979, *8*:715–32.

9. Diehl, H., and Mannerberg, D. Hypertension, hyperlipidaemia, angina, and coronary heart disease. In *Western Diseases: Their Emergence and Prevention,* Trowell, H. D., and Burkitt, D. P. eds. Cambridge: Harvard Univ. Press, 1981, p. 400.

10. Grundy, S. M. Saturated fats and coronary heart disease. In *Nutrition and the Killer Diseases,* Winick, M., ed. New York: Wiley, 1981, p. 76.

11. Pearce, M. L., and Dayton, S. Incidence of cancer in men on a diet high in polyunsaturated fat. *Lancet, I*:464–67.

12. Dayton, S., Pearce, M. L., Hashimoto, S., Dixon, W. J., and Tomi-yusua, U. A controlled clinical trial of a diet high in unsaturated fat in preventing complications of atherosclerosis. *Circulation,* 1969, *40*:Suppl. 2, 1–63.

13. National Research Council, Committee on Diet, Nutrition, and Cancer. *Diet, Nutrition, and Cancer.* Washington, D.C.: National Acad. Sci. 1982, pp. 5/20–21.

14. Barnard, R. J., Lattimore, L., Holly, R. G., Cherny, S., and Pritikin, N. Response of non-insulin-dependent diabetic patients to an intensive program of diet and exercise. *Diabetes Cure,* 1972, *5*:370–74.

15. Barnard, R. J., Guzy, P. M., Rosenberg, J. M., and O'Brien, L. T. Effects of an intensive exercise and nutrition program on patients with coronary artery disease: five-year follow-up (Abstract). *Med. Sci. Sports Exercise,* (1982), *14*:179.

Recipe Index